Unstable Angina
Diagnosis
and Management

P9-DDI-917

Commentary on the Agency for Health Care Policy and Research Clinical
Practice Guideline #10

Editor:

Michael H. Crawford, M.D.
Robert S. Flinn Professor
Chief, Division of Cardiology
University of New Mexico
Health Sciences Center

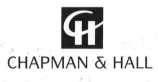

CHAPMAN & HALL

I(T)P® International Thomson Publishing

New York • Albany • Bonn • Boston • Cincinnati • Detroit • London • Madrid • Melbourne
Mexico City • Pacific Grove • Paris • San Francisco • Singapore • Tokyo • Toronto • Washington

JOIN US ON THE INTERNET
WWW: http://www.thomson.com
EMAIL: findit@kiosk.thomson.com
thomson.com is the on-line portal for the products, services and resources
available from International Thomson Publishing (ITP).
This Internet kiosk gives users immediate access to more than 34 ITP publishers and over
20,000 products. Through *thomson.com* Internet users can search catalogs, examine subject-
specific resource centers and subscribe to electronic discussion lists. You can purchase ITP
products from your local bookseller, or directly through *thomson.com.*

Visit Chapman & Hall's Internet Resource Center for information on our new publicatins, links to
useful sites on the World Wide Web and an opportunity to join our e-mail mailing list.
Point your browser to: **http://www.chaphall.com/** or **http://www.chaphall.com/chaphall/med.html** for
Medicine

Cover Design: Andrea Meyer, emDASH, Inc.
Copyright © 1997 Chapman & Hall

A service of **I**(**T**)**P**®

Printed in the United States of America

For more information, contact:

Chapman & Hall
115 Fifth Avenue
New York, NY 10003

Thomas Nelson Australia
102 Dodds Street
South Melbourne, 3205
Victoria, Australia

International Thomson Editores
Campos Eliseos 385, Piso 7
Col. Polanco
11560 Mexico D.F.
Mexico

International Thomson Publishing Asia
221 Henderson Road #05-10
Henderson Building
Singapore 0315

Chapman & Hall
2-6 Boundary Row
London SE1 8HN
England

Chapman & Hall GmbH
Postfach 100 263
D-69442 Weinheim
Germany

International Thomson Publishing-Japan
Hirakawacho-cho Kyowa Building, 3F
1-2-1 Hirakawacho-cho
Chiyoda-ku, 102 Tokyo
Japan

All rights reserved. No part of this work covered by the copyright hereon may be reproduced or used in any form or
by any means graphic, electronic, or mechanical, including photocopying, recording, taping, or information storage
and retrieval systems without the written permission of the publisher.

1 2 3 4 5 6 7 8 9 10 XXX 01 00 99 98 97

Original material from Braunwald E, Mark DB, Jones RH et al. Unstable Angina: Diagnosis and Management.
Clinical Practice Guideline Number 10 (amended) AHCPR Publication No. 94-0602. Rockville, MD: Agency for
Health Care Policy and Research and the National Heart, Lung, and Blood Institute, Public Health Service, U.S.
Department of Health and Human Services. May 1994.

Library of Congress Cataloging-in-Publication Data

Crawford, Michael H., 1943–
     Unstable angina : diagnosis and management: commentary on the Agency for Health Care Policy and
Research Clinical practice guidelines #10, Michael H. Crawford.
       p.   cm.—(Clinical practice guidelines series)
     Includes bibliographical references and index.
     ISBN 0-412-09771-0 (alk. paper)
     1. Angina pectoris. I. United States. Agency for Health Care Policy and Research. II. Title.
III. Series [DNLM: 1. Unstable angina. 2. Angina, Unstable—diagnosis 3. Angina, Unstable—therapy.
WG 298 C899u 1996]
RC685.A6C73   1996
616.1'22—dc20
DNLM/DLC
for Library of Congress
                                                                                                96-26865
                                                                                                CIP

British Library Cataloguing in Publication Data available

To order this or any other Chapman & Hall book, please contact **International Thomson Publishing**, **7625
Empire Drive, Florence, KY 41042**. Phone: (606) 525-6600 or 1-800-842-3636.
Fax: (606) 525-7778, e-mail: order@chaphall.com.

For a complete listing of Chapman & Hall's titles, send your requests to
Chapman & Hall, Dept. BC, 115 Fifth Avenue, New York, NY 10003.

Contents

TABLES

FIGURES

Preface

The AHCPR committee that developed these clinical practice guidelines on unstable angina did an excellent job reviewing the current literature and expert opinions, and formulating this practical approach to a complex, potentially high risk area of heart disease management. The guidelines help the clinician more effectively manage patients to the benefit of the patients and the physician (litigation avoidance). Also, they occasion a re-evaluation of certain costly practices that may or may not be necessary in all patients, such as hospital admission. Unstable angina is a frequent admission diagnosis that managed care organizations are scrutinizing carefully. The guidelines give the physician information of value for developing reasonable admission criteria and parameters for the application of various testing strategies and treatments. Thus, attention to these guidelines should benefit all—patients, physicians and health care systems.

The purpose of this publication is to reprint the guidelines with an index (not available in the Government's version) and to provide expert commentary designed to mitigate some of the weaknesses of the guideline format. These weaknesses include: 1) a pedantic style that does not include clinical examples; 2) a tendency toward conservatism because of the committee consensus necessity; 3) a fiscally conservative approach reflecting the sponsoring organization's bias toward cost cutting; and 4) a lack of consideration of new data since 1993 because of the March 1994 publication date.

Also, the guidelines assume that increased risks of adverse events in patients is acceptable in order to contain costs, as long as they are within reason. Unfortunately our legal system is not based upon this premise, but rather that any adverse outcome is someone's fault and they are legally liable under Tort law. The someone is most often the physician. Due to peculiarities in ERISA legislation,

HMO, who dictate certain conservative practices as a condition of continued employment, can pass the risk to the physician. Thus, until there is meaningful Tort reform and changes in ERISA laws, it is only fair to point out to physicians areas where explicitly following the guidelines may put them at odds with currently accepted medical practice. Although the guidelines may help them ultimately prevail in a court case, most physicians would rather avoid litigation.

Reading any practice guideline should be an educational experience. These guidelines are no exception as the committee has carefully referenced and described much of the important literature in this area. We have designed our comments to augment the educational value of the guidelines by including the most recent papers and increasing the discussion in critical areas. Finally, all the algorithms are repeated at the end of the book on cards that can be torn out and used for quick reference.

We believe that this publication will provide the best of both worlds—an indexed reprinting of an excellent guideline and a practical interpretation of the most recent thinking on the management of unstable angina patients. Also, this book will bring the reader up to date in the area of acute ischemic heart disease syndromes, permitting an assimilation of new knowledge in the proper perspective of what is already known.

Michael H. Crawford, M.D., Editor

Robert S. Flinn Professor, Chief, Division of Cardiology,
University of New Mexico, Health Sciences Center

Contributors Providing Commentary

Michael H. Crawford, M.D.
Robert S. Flinn Professor
Chief of Cardiology
University of New Mexico School of Medicine
Albuquerque, New Mexico

Bruce K. Shively, M.D.
Associate Professor of Medicine
Director of Cardiac Non-invasive Laboratories
University of New Mexico School of Medicine
Albuquerque, New Mexico

T. Craig Timm, M.D.
Assistant Professor of Medicine
Director, Cardiac Catheterization Laboratory
University Hospital
University of New Mexico School of Medicine
Albuquerque, New Mexico

Guideline Development and Use

Guidelines are systematically developed statements to assist practitioner and patient decisions about appropriate health care for specific clinical conditions. This guideline was developed by a private-sector panel convened by the Agency for Health Care Policy and Research (AHCPR) and the National Heart, Lung, and Blood Institute (NHLBI). The panel, with the assistance of Duke University Medical Center, employed an explicit, science-based methodology and expert clinical judgment to develop specific statements on patient assessment and management of unstable angina.

Extensive literature searches were conducted, and critical reviews and syntheses were used to evaluate empirical evidence and significant outcomes. Peer review and field review were undertaken to evaluate the validity and utility of the guideline in clinical practice. The panel's recommendations are primarily based on the published scientific literature. When the scientific literature was incomplete or inconsistent in a particular area, the recommendations reflect the professional justment of panel members and consultants.

The guideline reflects the state of knowledge, current at the time of publication, on effective and appropriate care. Given the inevitable changes in the state of scientific information and technology, periodic review, updating, and revision will be done.

We believe that the AHCPR-and NHLBI-assisted clinical practice guideline will make positive contributions to the quality of care in the United States. We encourage practitioners and patients to use the information provided in the guideline. The recommendations may not be appropriate for use in all circumstances. Decisions to adopt any particular recommendation must be made by the practitioner in light of a available resources and circumstances presented by individual patients.

J. Jarrett Clinton, MD
Administrator
Agency for Health Care
Policy and Research

Claude Lenfant, MD
Director
National Heart, Lung,
and Blood Institute

Publication of this guideline does not necessarily represent endorsement by the U.S. Department of Health and Human Services.

Clinical Practice Guideline

Number 10

Unstable Angina: Diagnosis and Management

Eugene Braunwald, MD, Chairman
Daniel B. Mark, MD, MPH
Robert H. Jones, MD
Melvin D. Cheitlin, MD
Valentin Fuster, MD, PhD
Kathleen M. McCauley, PhD, RN, CS
Conan Edwards, PhD
Lee A. Green, MD, MPH
Alvin I. Mushlin, MD, ScM
Julie A. Swain, MD
Earl E. Smith III, MD
Marie Cowan, RN, MS, PhD
Gregory C. Rose, MD
Craig A. Concannon, MD
Cindy L. Grines, MD
Leslie Brown, MPH, JD
Bruce W. Lytle, MD
Lee Goldman, MD
Eric J. Topol, MD
James T. Willerson, MD
Jay Brown, MD
Nancy Archibald, MHA, MBA

U.S. Department of Health and Human Services
Public Health Service
Agency for Health Care Policy and Research
National Heart, Lung, and Blood Institute

AHCPR Publication No. 94-0602

Panel Members

Eugene Braunwald, MD
(Panel Chair)
Hersey Professor of the Theory and
Practice of Medicine
Chairman, Department of Medicine
Harvard Medical School
Brigham & Women's Hospital
Boston, MA

Jay Brown, MD (Deceased)
Chief, Division of Cardiology
Harlem Hospital Center
Clinical Associate Professor of
Medicine
Columbia University
College of Physicians and Surgeons
New York, NY

Leslie Brown, MPH, JD
Deputy Director
Division of Adult Health Promotion
Department of Environment, Health,
and Natural Resources
State of North Carolina
Raleigh, NC

Melvin D, Cheitlin, MD
Chief, Cardiology Division
San Francisco General Hospital
Professor of Medicine
University of California, San
Francisco
School of Medicine
San Francisco, CA

Craig A. Concannon, MD
Chief of Staff
Mitchell County Hospital
Clinical Professor
University of Kansas School of
Medicine, Wichita
Wichita, KS

Marie Cowan, RN, MS, PhD
Associate Dean of Research and
Practice
Professor of Physiological Nursing
University of Washington School of
Nursing
Seattle, WA

Conan Edwards, PhD
Volunteer
American Association of Retired
Persons
Madison, WI

Valentin Fuster, MD, PhD
Arthur M. and Hilda A. Master
Professor of Medicine
Director, Cardiovascular Institute
Vice Chairman, Department of
Medicine
Mount Sinai Medical Center
Boston, MA

Lee Goldman, MD
Professor of Medicine
Harvard Medical School
Chief Medical Officer
Brigham & Women's Hospital
Boston, MA

Lee A. Green, MD, MPH
Assistant Professor
Department of Family Practice
University of Michigan
Medical School
Lecturer in Health Services
Management and Policy
University of Michigan School of
Public Health
Ann Arbor, MI

Cindy L. Grines, MD
Director
Cardiac Catheterization Laboratory

William Beaumont Hospital
Royal Oak, MI

Bruce W. Lytle, MD
Surgeon
Department of Thoracic and
Cardiovascular Surgery
Cleveland Clinic Foundation
Cleveland, OH

**Kathleen M. McCauley, PhD,
RN, CS**
Assistant Professor of Cardiovascular
Nursing
University of Pennsylvania School of
Nursing
Cardiovascular Clinical Specialist
Hospital of the University of
Pennsylvania
Philadelphia, PA

Alvin I. Mushlin, MD, ScM
Professor of Community Medicine
and Medicine
University of Rochester Medical
Center
Rochester, NY

Gregory C. Rose, MD
Director, Mobile Cardiac Care Unit
Wake Medical Center
Raleigh, NCEarl E. Smith III, MD
Medical Director and Chief
Emergency Department Erlanger
Medical Center

Clinical Instructor
Department of Medicine Chattanooga
Unit
University of Tennessee College of
Medicine
Chattanooga, TN

Julie A. Swain, MD
Chief, Division of Cardiovascular
Surgery
Vice Chairman, Department of
Surgery
University of Nevada
School of Medicine, Las Vegas
Las Vegas, NV

Eric J. Topol, MD
Professor of Medicine
Cleveland Clinic Health Sciences
Center
Ohio State University Chairman,
Department of Cardiology
Cleveland Clinic Foundation
Cleveland, OH

James T. Willerson, MD
Edward Randall III Professor
Chairman, Department of Internal
Medicine
University of Texas Health Science
Center, Houston Medical Director
Texas Heart Institute
Houston, TX

Duke University Participants

Project Oversight

Robert H. Jones, MD
Project Director
Mary and Deryl Hart
Professor of Surgery

Daniel B. Mark, MD, MPH
Project Co-Director
Author/Editor
Associate Professor
Division of Cardiology

Nancy Archibald, MHA, MBA
Project Manager

Vanessa Moore
Staff Assistant
Stastical Analysis

L. Richard Smith, PhD
Biostatistician
Assistant Professor
Division of Experimental Surgery

Karen Kesler, MS
Biostatistician

Consultants

Robert M. Califf, MD
Associate Professor
Division of Cardiology
Director, Cardiac Care Unit

David B. Pryor, MD
Associate Professor
Division of Cardiology
Literature Review

David B. Matchar, MD
Methodologist
Associate Professor
Director, Center for Health Policy
Research and Education

Robert H. Sprinkle, MD, PhD
Assistant Professor
Literature Review Manager
Center for Health Policy Research and
Education

Victor Hassellblad, PhD
Statistician/Meta-analyst
Associate Professor
Center for Health Policy Research and
Education

Leslee Shaw, PhD
Reviewer

Computer Support

Donald F. Fortin, MD
Medical Consultant
Assistant Professor
Division of Cardiology Director,
Cardiac
Imaging Center

J. Douglass Hanemann
Technical Consultant

Although the guideline is based on the Committee's assessment of the medical literature, the opinion of the Committee members is relied upon heavily. Interestingly, not all of the Committee members are physicians. Of the 19 members, 9 are general cardiologists, 4 are general physicians, 2 are interventional cardiologists, 2 are nurses, 1 is a lawyer, and 1 is a layperson. In addition, there was a group at Duke University who provided literature review, computer support, statistical analysis, and general consultation. This group included 9 physicians, of which 5 were cardiologists or cardiovascular surgeons.

FOREWORD

Unstable angina is a transitory clinical syndrome usually associated with an increased tempo or intensity of symptoms that are thought to be indicative of coronary artery disease accompanied by an increased risk of cardiac death and myocardial infarction. This common condition accounts for a significant amount of disability and death. In 1991 alone, the National Center for Health Statistics reported 570,000 hospitalizations for this condition, resulting in 3.1 million hospital days.

This Clinical Practice Guideline provides recommendations and supporting evidence for all aspects of the diagnosis and treatment of unstable angina in both the inpatient and outpatient settings. The management of patients with acute myodarcial infarction or stable angina is addressed only when these related conditions border indistinguishably with unstable angina. The panel assumes that medical practitioners will use general medical knowledge and clinical judgment in flexibly applying the general principles and specific recommendations of this document to the management of individual patients with unstable angina.

The guideline is written to be directly applicable to patient care. An initial chapter defines and provides background information about unstable angina. Subsequent chapters outline patient management in seven discrete phases: initial evaluation and treatment, outpatient care, intensive medical management, nonintensive medical management, noninvasive testing, cardiac catheterization and myocardial revascularization, and hospital discharge care. Chapter organization reflects common stages of care determined by requirements for specialized facilities and personnel but is not meant to constrain a management sequence for all patients. Appropriate chapters should be applied as patients enter, exit, or re-enter specific phases of their illness. The goal of patient counseling sections included in each chapter is to foster a sense of partnership and reasonable expectation between the patient and patient advocate and the health care team.

The diagnosis of unstable angina implies risk of cardiac injury and death. Needlessly overcautious management strategies initiated in attempt to eliminate all risks often spawn secondary risks and are discouraged both for this reason and because of the extra cost burden they impose. Diagnostic and therapeutic strategies recommended are those most likely to maximize benefits given the current state of medical knowledge. However, adherence to this or any other guideline will not ensure perfect medical outcomes. Application of the most carefully reasoned clinical judgment based on current medical knowledge cannot eliminate all risk in the management of patients with unstable angina.

This section clearly states the mission of the guideline: to discourage "needlessly overcautious management strategies initiated in an attempt to eliminate all risks" of unstable angina. Two rationales are given for this mission. The first is to prevent secondary risks of these management strategies. Here they are obviously referring to the risks of cardiac catheterization and revascularization. The second rationale is to reduce costs. Clearly, the biggest consumer of costs in any illness is hospitalization expense. So, immediately, the physician appreciates that the guideline will discourage hospitalization, cardiac catheterization, and revascularization of unstable angina patients. In fact, the guideline goes to great lengths to detail who needs hospitalization and who needs cardiac catheterization and revascularization. The guideline authors believe that it is impossible to eliminate all risks, so the physician must use "reasoned clinical judgment based upon current medical knowledge." What they are referring to is so-called evidence-based medicine or the practice of medicine based upon the medical literature. The guideline relies heavily on the medical literature for its recommendations. Since the medical literature is continuously growing this means that the guideline was out of date the day it was published and its timeliness worsens with time. As we will point out in these comments the publication of certain recent studies has made some of the guideline recommendations obsolete. Most of the recent studies support a more aggressive approach than recommended by this guideline.

Abstract

Recommendations on the care of patients with unstable angina made this clinical practice guideline are based on a combination of evidence obtained through extensive literature reviews and, in cases where evidence was lacking, on the consensus opinions of the expert panel. Principal conclusions of this guideline include:

- Many patients suspected of having unstable angia can be discharged home after adequete initial evaluation.
- Further outpatient evaluation of patients with symptoms of unstable angina judged at initial evaluation to be at low risk for complications should be concluded within 72 hours after initial presentation.
- Patients with unstable angina judged to be at intermediate or high risk of complications should receive aspirin, heparin, nitroglycerin, and beta-blocker therapy and should be hospitalized for careful monitoring of their clinical course.
- Intravenous thrombolytic therapy should not be administered to patients without evidence of acute myocardial infarction.

This abstract is a summary of the major points of the guideline. Clearly, the conclusion of the guideline is that we must discourage the aggressive therapeutic approach of hospitalization and cardiac catheterization for all patients with unstable angina, and that we must accept some risk of events to contain costs.

- Assessment of prognosis by noninvasive testing often aids selection of appropriate therapy.
- Coronary angiography is appropriate for patients judged to be at high risk for cardiac complications or death based on their clinical course or results of noninvasive testing.
- Coronary artery bypass surgery should be recommended for almost all patients with left main disease and many patients with three-vessel disease especially those with left ventricular dysfunction.
- The discharge care plan should include continued monitoring of symptoms, approprate drug therapy including aspirin and risk-factor modification, and counseling.

EXECUTIVE SUMMARY

Purpose

The purpose of this guideline is to define diagnostic and management strategies likely to maximize therapeutic benefit for patients with unstable angina. Recommendations are expected to be flexibly applied to individual patients by informed practitioners using reasonable clinical judgments.

The purpose of this executive summary is to describe the process of guideline development and provide an overview of its scope and content. Clinicians desiring a summary of this guideline, designed to guide actions during actual patient management, may wish to obtain the companion document designed for this purpose, *Quick Reference Guide for Clinicians, Number 10, Diagnosing and Managing Unstable Angina,* which is available upon request from the Agency for Health Care Policy and Research (AHCPR).

Process of Guideline Development

This clinical practice guideline on the diagnosis and management of unstable angina was developed by a private-sector panel of emergency, family, and internal medicine specialists; cardiologists; cardiac surgeons; nurses; and consumer and public health representatives. The panel was convened and supported by AHCPR and the National Heart, Lung, and Blood Institute (NHLBI). The panel was assisted in all aspects of its work by a professional staff from Duke University.

Using the National Library of Medicine's medical subject headings, staff conducted a search of available data bases which yielded over 5,000 abstracts relating to unstable angina. Nearly 2,500 relevant articles were organized by an outline of topics related to the usual management steps in patients with unstable angina. Review of topically ordered abstracts identified 130 randomized clinical trials, 319 clinical studies of excellent quality, and 1,351 clinical studies of good quality which were analyzed for appropriateness of methodology and summarized for panel review. Only results of published studies and studies known to be accepted for publication were considered in reaching panel recommendations. However, the text of the guideline refers in general terms to findings of a small number of major randomized trials which have recently been presented at national meetings. The trials are mentioned because information available at the time of their publication will likely influence management decisions in patients with unstable angina.

Studies on topics corresponding to individual guideline recommendations were reviewed together, and the overall quality of scientific evidence available was graded A, B, or C. A strength of evidence = A grade required at least one randomized controlled trial as part of the body of literature of overall good quality and consistency addressing the specific recommendation. A strength of evidence = B grade required availability of well-conducted clinical studies but no randomized clinical trials on the topic of the recommendation. A strength of evidence = C grade indicated absence of directly applicable clinical studies of good quality.

These recommendations were made by panel consensus using related information, general principles of medical care, and clinical experience. An informal process of group discussion was used to achieve panel consensus on the language and strength of evidence of each recommendation.

Evidence was poor or lacking to assist panel deliberation on many aspects of diagnosing and managing unstable angina, and the quality of available scientific evidence did not always relate to the clinical importance of the topic. Therefore, the language used in each recommendation reflects the perceived importance of the statement in patient care, and the strength of evidence grade reflects the body of scientific literature available to support the recommendation. The guideline was revised to reflect the thoughtful comments of 75 individuals representing 24 professional peer organizations with interest and expertise in unstable angina. The guideline was reviewed and tested by 44 practitioners for practicality and reasonableness in clinical practice.

Definition of Unstable Angina

Throughout this guideline, unstable angina is defined as having three possible presentations: symptoms of angina at rest (usually prolonged >20 minutes), new onset (<2 months) exertional angina of at least Canadian Cardiovascular Society Classification (CCSC) class III in severity, or recent (<2 months) acceleration of angina as reflected by an increase in severity of at least one CCSC class to at least CCSC class III. In most, but not all, of these patients, symptoms will be caused by significant coronary artery disease (CAD). Variant angina, non-Q-wave myocardial infarction (MI), and post-MI (>24 hours) angina are part of the spectrum of unstable angina.

Diagnosis of Unstable Angina

A diagnosis of unstable angina requires determination of the likelihood of CAD and assessment of the severity of presentation. The likelihood of significant CAD in patients presenting with acute chest pain syndrome is related to the physician's assessment of the patient's symptoms as angina, categorized as definite, probable, probably not, or definitely not angina; evidence of prior MI or other indicators of CAD; and the sex, age, and number of major risk factors for atherosclerosis. Other factors important in diagnosis of unstable angina include a known history of variant angina or cocaine use and details of prior treatment for known or suspected CAD. Physical findings of value include a transient S_3 or S_4 mitral regurgitation (MR) murmur or precordial lift during an episode of discomfort. The presence of bruits or pulse deficits suggesting extracardiac vascular disease increases the likelihood of CAD.

The standard 12-lead electrocardiogram (ECG) provides crucial information in the diagnosis of unstable angina, and recordings during periods of both pain and absence of pain are useful. Markers of high likelihood of CAD on ECG include ST-segment elevation or depression ≥ 1mm, deep symmetrical T-wave inversion in multiple precordial leads, or any transient ECG change occurring during pain. ST-segment depression ≥0.5 mm but <1 mm, T-wave inversion ≥1 mm in leads with dominant R-waves, and nonspecific ST- and T-wave changes are features of patients with an intermediate likelihood of CAD. These clinical features on initial evaluation can be used to stratify patients into high, intermediate, and low likelihood of CAD.

Prognosis of Unstable Angina

Risk of death or ischemic complications in patients with unstable angina is lower than with MI but higher than with stable angina. This risk is greater when symptoms first occur and declines rapidly to baseline levels, defined by characteristics of patients with stable angina, within about 2 months of initial presentation. The prognosis of patients presenting with symptoms suggestive of unstable angina is determined by the likelihood of CAD, the tempo of the recent clinical course, and by factors that affect the likelihood that a patient will survive should an acute ischemic event occur. Important historic elements to define the tempo of presentation of symptoms include the current frequency and change in frequency and severity of angina over the recent time prior to presentation. Prolonged episodes of severe chest pain are important markers of high-risk unstable angina. The important prognostic elements on physical examination include any evidence of acute congestive heart failure (CHF), a new or worsening MR murmur, or systemic hypotension, particularly during an episode of severe pain. ECG findings suggesting increased risk are dynamic shifts in ST-segment change with ≥1 mm of ST-segment depression or elevation or T-wave inversions that resolve when symptoms are relieved. Through the use of these characteristics, patients with the diagnosis of unstable angina can be stratified into three groups characterized as having a low, intermediate, or high risk of death or nonfatal MI. As patients progress through the clinical course of their disease, additional events (such as an assessment of left ventricular [LV] ejection fraction [EF]) may be obtained that permit the assessment of prognosis to be updated or refined.

Guideline Recommendations

Patient Counseling

The panel recommends informing and involving the patient and his or her family or advocate in all important care decisions. Sufficient information describing diagnosis, prognosis, and treatment options should be given to patients to permit them to choose care alternatives they prefer.

Initial Evaluation and Treatment of Patients with Unstable Angina

Because the diagnosis of unstable angina can be quite difficult, initial evaluation of patients with symptoms consistent with ischemic pain should usually take place in a medical facility with the capability of performing an ECG, not over the telephone. In general, patients with ongoing pain should be evaluated initially in an emergency department (ED) with the capability of providing ECG monitoring, advanced cardiac life support (ACLS), intravenous (IV) pharmacologic therapy, and radiographic examinations. Patients without ongoing pain may be evaluated initially in outpatient facilities with diagnostic probabilities and evaluate the short-term risk of death and other major complications. The results of this evaluation will set the pace of further care and form the basis of the working diagnosis. The two goals of initial management of patients with unstable angina are to institute immediate therapy and move the patient to a proper environment for the monitoring of complications. In many cases, stabilization progresses concurrently with patient evaluation.

Initial evaluation should be complete and treatment begun within an hour of presentation to the ED. All patients with unstable angina should receive aspirin (ASA) unless they have documented hypersensitivity or active bleeding. Those with persistent symptoms or ECG changes suggesting ongoing ischemia should also receive nitroglycerin (NTG). Beta blockers and IV heparin are indicated for patients with intermediate- and high-risk unstable angina who do not have contraindications to these drugs. Unless patients have a compelling history for acute MI accompanied by ST-segment evaluation or left bundle branch block (LBBB) on the 12-lead ECG, IV thrombolytic therapy is not indicated.

Patients with unstable angina and high-risk features with persistent ischemia or hemodynamic instability should be admitted to an ICU, intermediate care unit, or other cardiac care environment. All high-risk patients and many intermediate-risk patients should have serial cardiac enzymes and ECGs to exclude the possibility of acute MI. Low-risk patients can be further evaluated and managed as outpatients. Patients with acute MI with indications for thrombolytic or other reperfusion therapy, patients with stable angina, and patients considered not to have CAD are excluded from this guideline at the conclusion of initial evaluation.

Outpatient Care

Patients judged to be at low risk when initially seen who, therefore, are not admitted to a medical facility, should have a thorough evaluation scheduled within 72 hours if a definitive evaluation cannot be completed at the time of initial presentation. At the time of subsequent evaluation, attention is directed toward further assessing the cause of the patient's symptoms, evaluating the risk of future adverse cardiac events, and providing adequate symptom relief.

Patients considered not to have CAD after this evaluation should be reassured that their symptoms are very unlikely to be due to CAD and should be evaluated appropriately to determine the cause of the symptoms. The care of patients thought to have CAD should match the severity of the process. Most patients will require some pharmacologic therapy to relieve symptoms. In addition, exercise or pharmacologic stress testing will usually be a part of this detailed workup. All patients should receive information on the modification of CAD risk factors.

xxiv *Unstable Angina: Diagnosis and Management*

Intensive Medical Management

Patients considered to have ongoing manifestations of unstable angina should receive intensive medical management. The goals of this phase of care are to relieve pain and ischemia and to prevent the progression of the underlying disease process to MI or death. ASA, heparin, nitrates, and beta blockers begun at the time of initial evaluation should be titrated to a dosage adequate to relieve ischemia but avoid hemodynamic compromise. Morphine sulfate may be necessary to help relieve severe anginal symptoms that have not resolved with initial therapy. Calcium channel blockers should not be used as initial therapy but can be added to the regimen of patients who are unable to tolerate nitrates or beta blockers or in whom these agents were not effective. Calcium channel blockers should not be given to patients with pulmonary edema or evidence of LV dysfunction. Aggressive medical management can control the presenting symptoms of most patients with unstable angina.

Careful monitoring of patients for recurrent ischemia should continue after the desired level of medical therapy has been reached. The presence of recurrent symptoms may indicate a need for a more intensive medical regimen or triage to early cardiac catheterization and revascularization. Unless complications of ischemia are noted, an optimal medical regimen should be pursued for ≥24 hours before declaring it a failure. However, to use this time as an absolute requirement in the case of every patient would be inappropriate or even dangerous. Generally, if anginal symptoms persist for >1 hour after aggressive medical therapy, which includes ASA, heparin, IV nitrates, and beta blockers, the patient should be re-evaluated more comprehensively to be sure there are no unaddressed precipitating factors, reconsider the possibility of noncoronary diseases that may mimic unstable angina, and reaffirm that the most appropriate diagnosis remains unstable angina and not acute MI or other more serious illness.

Progression to Nonintensive Medical Management

Patients with high- or intermediate-risk unstable angina whose symptoms have been controlled for 24 hours with intensive medical management will have progressed to a lower risk phase and are appropriate for nonintensive medical management. Patients with intermediate or low risk may be admitted directly into this phase after initial evaluation in the ED. During nonintensive medical management, the emphasis shifts from acute stabilization to the design of a maintenance medical regimen that will suppress reactivation of acute disease activity. Failure of therapy at this phase of care is indicated by recurrent angina refractory to treatment for >20 minutes or recurring more than once on nonparenteral medication. These patients are expected to return to intensive medical management. Other objectives of care often include optimization of the therapeutic regimen and noninvasive testing for risk stratifaction.

Noninvasive Testing

Important management decisions in patients with unstable angina revolve around ongoing risk stratification. In some patients the early clinical course will be characterized by recurrent ECG-documented ischemia. In other patients further evaluation will suggest that the initial diagnosis of unstable angina may have been incorrect. These patients, who are recognized by clinical presentation to have such a high or low probability of high-risk CAD that further risk stratification by noninvasive testing would not alter management, and patients whose other comorbid conditions make stress testing unnecessary or inappropriate have no need to undergo noninvasive testing. Unless cardiac catheterization is indicated, all other patients hospitalized for unstable angina should undergo noninvasive testing after stabilization has been achieved and prior to discharge or as soon as possible thereafter. In this context, noninvasive testing is most useful to assess the adequacy of current therapy, estimate prognosis, and guide decisions on further evaluation and management.

Cardiac Catheterization and Myocardial Revascularization

Common indications for cardiac catheterization in patients with unstable angina include: (1) failure to stabilize with adequate medical therapy; (2) recurrent unstable angina; (3) high-risk result of noninvasive test; (4) prior revascularization procedure; and (5) diagnosis or exclusion of significant CAD in patients with multiple clinical episodes of unstable angina without objective documentation of ischemia. Individual patient characteristics and preferences should temper application of these general indications to specific clinical situations.

The goal of cardiac catheterization in patients with unstable angina is to provide detailed structural information necessary to assess prognosis and select an appropriate long-term management strategy. The procedure is usually helpful in choosing between medical therapy, percutaneous transluminal coronary angioplasty (PTCA), or coronary artery bypass graft (CABG) surgery in patients with unstable angina who remain at significant risk for future cardiac events. Patients with extensive comorbidity felt not to be suitable for revascularization and patients who do not wish to consider interventional therapy should not undergo diagnostic catheterization.

Patients found at catheterization to have significant left main disease ($\geq$50%) or significant ($\geq$70%) three-vessel disease with depressed LV function (EF <0.50) should undergo CABG to improve survival as well as relieve symptoms. Patients with two- or three-vessel disease with proximal severe subtotal stenosis ($\geq$95%) of the left anterior descending coronary artery (LAD) may also experience a survival benefit from revascularization. Other patients are appropriately treated for control of anginal symptoms by CABG, PTCA, or medical therapy.

Hospital Discharge and Postdischarge Care

Patients responding to intensive and nonintensive medical therapy and patients undergoing CABG or PTCA during their admission should be instructed on appropriate activities after hospital discharge. Discharge plans should include provisions for clinical followup and risk-factor modification. Continued long-term management of the patient with unstable angina should include ASA therapy indefinitely unless contraindicated. Patients who have stable symptoms at followup may be managed as if they have stable angina.

Overview

Commentary by Michael H. Crawford, M.D.

Definition of Terms and Processes

Readers of this guideline who are not regularly involved in the management of patients with unstable angina should refer to the list of acronyms and glossary of medical terminology included with this guideline and the list of essential definitions on page 133. However, even experienced clinicians will enhance their understanding and use of subsequent chapters in this document by a review of terms used to describe CAD presentations that are often blurred in common clinical usage. The authors of this guideline propose the following definitions in discussing the management of patients with unstable angina.

Definition of Unstable Angina

Throughout this guideline, unstable angina is broadly defined as a clinical syndrome that falls between stable angina and acute MI in the spectrum of presentations of CAD (Braunwald, 1989). The intent of the definition is to include all patients with acute presentations of CAD with the exclusion of only those patients with reperfusion-eligible acute MI. In most, but not all, of these patients, these symptoms will be caused by significant CAD. Since an adequate operational definition of unstable angina for this guideline must be based on the information available at the time of the initial presentation and evaluation, patients with a spectrum of underlying problems may receive a clinical diagnosis of unstable angina until additional diagnostic information becomes available (e.g., cardiac enzymes, noninvasive testing, or results of cardiac catheterization). The three principal presentations of unstable angina are listed in Table 1.

By design, this operational definition includes patients who will subsequently be found to have had an acute MI, as well as patients who will subsequently be found not to have significant coronary disease. The Canadian Cardiovascular Society classification (CCSC) system is used throughout this guideline to grade the severity of anginal pain and discomfort (see Table 2).

Definition of Care Environments
Table 3 summarizes characteristics of five common clinical care environments for patients with unstable angina.

Definition of Strength of Evidence Grading
The strength of evidence grade for each recommendation within this guideline is followed by a brief discussion of the underlying rationale. Individual studies received ratings based on experimental design and overall quality. Randomized controlled trials received the highest ratings, other well-designed studies received a lower score, and studies with design or methodologic deficiencies received the lowest rating. The strength of evidence for each recommendation is summarized as an A, B, or C rating which most closely characterizes the total scientific literature available to address the topic (see Table 4).

Often, the most basic patient management questions and the most well-accepted care strategies are the most difficult to test. For example, no randomized clinical trials are likely to be conducted to evaluate the importance of a medical history and physical examination in patients with unstable angina. Therefore, the strength of evidence grade does not always reflect the importance of the recommendation to patient care. The specific language used to formulate each recommendation conveys panel opinion of both the clinical importance attributed to the topic and the strength of evidence available.

Background Information on Unstable Angina
Proper application of the action-oriented recommendations made in this guideline assumes understanding of the basic disease process and familiarity with the common clinical presentation of patients with unstable angina. The background information in this section provides an overview of the principles necessary to place the recommendations in subsequent chapters in a balanced clinical context.

Unstable Angina in the Spectrum of Coronary Artery Disease
CAD is the most important cause of death and disability in the United States. Only about 10 percent of patients with CAD have unstable angina as their initial presentation if patients who experience an MI are retrospectively excluded. However, patients with established CAD (either chronic stable angina or prior MI) commonly cycle through unstable phases. As a clinical syndrome, unstable angina shares ill-defined borders with chronic stable angina, a presentation with lower risk, and with acute MI, a presentation with higher risk.

Unstable angina occurs in a variety of clinical scenarios, including in patients

Table 1. Three principal presentations of unstable angina

Rest angina	Angina occurring at rest and usually prolonged >20 minutes occurring within a week of presentation.
New onset angina	Angina of at least CCSC III severity with onset within 2 months of initial presentation.
Increasing angina	Previously diagnosed angina that is distinctly more frequent, longer in duration or lower in threshold (i.e., increased by at least one CCSC class within 2 months of initial presentation to at least CCSC III severity).

Note: CCSC = Canadian Cardiovascular Society classification.

Unstable angina, as defined by this guideline, is diagnosed when the physician first sees the patient and is based upon the information available at that time. Three independent criteria for the diagnosis are given. The first criterion is angina decubitus that lasts more than 20 minutes. This criterion includes variant angina, since in Western civilizations up to 75 percent of such patients have fixed CAD. The second criterion is new onset exertional angina of CCSC III or higher for less than 2 months. The Canadian system is an intuitive one based upon the physical limitations of the patient and is much like the New York Heart Association functional classification of heart failure patients. The guideline gives an excellent summary of the CCSC system (Table 2). The third criterion is recent acceleration of angina of at least one CCSC class to at least CCSC class III. The diagnosis of unstable angina assumes that the patient's symptoms are due to CAD in most cases. Also, it is assumed that since this diagnosis is an initial encounter diagnosis, a few patients will prove not to have CAD and some patients will later be diagnosed with MI. In fact, non-Q-wave MI and post-MI angina are included in the unstable angina clinical scenarios considered by this guideline.

Table 2. Grading of angina pectoris by the Canadian
Cardiovascular Society classification system

Class	Description of stage
Class I	Ordinary physical activity does not cause angina, such as walking, climbing stairs. Angina [occurs] with strenuous, rapid, or prolonged exertion at work or recreation.
Class II	Slight limitation of ordinary activity. Angina occurs on walking or climbing stairs rapidly, walking uphill, walking or stair climbing after meals, or in cold, or in wind, or under emotional stress, or only during the few hours after awakening. Walking more than two blocks on the level and climbing more than one flight of ordinary stairs at a normal pace and in normal condition.
Class III	Marked limitations of ordinary physical activity. Angina occurs on walking one to two blocks on the level and climbing one flight of stairs in normal conditions and at a normal pace.
Class IV	Inability to carry on any physical activity without discomfort—anginal symptoms may be present at rest.

Source: Campeau L. Grading of angina pectoris [letter].
Circulation, 54:522–523, 1976. Copyright 1976, American
Heart Association, Inc. Used with permission.

without known CAD, with prior stable CAD, soon after MI, and following myocardial revascularization by CABG or PTCA. Patients presenting with unstable angina may undergo any of the diagnostic and therapeutic procedures used for other CAD patients. Therefore, recommendations for the management of patients with unstable angina of necessity address questions pertinent to patients with any mode of presentation of CAD.

Despite the fact that death rates for CAD are decreasing (Gillum and Feinlieb, 1988; Feinlieb, 1984), hospital discharge rates for this disorder appear to have stabilized since 1979 (Feinlieb, Havlik, Gillum et al., 1989). The number of hospitalizations for which the principal diagnosis was unstable angina (ICD-9-CM

Table 3. Definition of unstable angina care environments

Emergency Department (ED)

To be considered an adequate ED for patients with unstable angina, a hospital or clinic
    entry point or emergency chest pain center should be continuously staffed by personnel
    competent in performing an ECG, initial evaluation and treatment of patients with
    unstable angina, cardiac monitoring, and advanced cardiac life support (ACLS). Such a
    facility should be able to provide routine laboratory testing and radiographic studies. In
    remote regions of the country, where continuous availability of trained personnel is not
    feasible, arrangement of consultation linkages with practitioners with appropriate
    training using facsimile and telephone communication is recommended.

Outpatient Facility

A doctor's office, hospital-associated or free-standing clinic, or other environment to be
    used for care of patients initially presenting with symptoms of unstable angina who are
    not hospitalized should have the capability to perform a 12-lead ECG and be staffed by
    personnel who are competent in placing a secure IV line and performing basic life
    support (BLS).

Intensive Care Unit (ICU)

This unit, which may also be called a coronary care unit (CCU), represents the highest
    level of medical intensive care available in a hospital. Typical characteristics include a
    nurse to patient ratio of 1:1 or 1:2; cardiac monitoring; immediate access to persons
    trained in ACLS; and capabilities for arterial line and pulmonary artery catheter
    placement, temporary pacemaker placement, and mechanical ventilation. Some, but not
    all, such units will have facilities for intra-aortic balloon placement. This unit can
    handle all forms of vasoactive continuous IV infusion. Nurses are competent in the
    recognition and treatment of arrhythmias and evaluation of ischemic symptoms.

Intermediate Care Unit

This unit, which may also be referred to as a cardiac monitoring or step-down unit, has a
    lower nurse to patient ratio, typically 1:3 to 1:5, than an ICU. It can provide continuous
    ECG monitoring and prompt access to personnel trained in ACLS. Personnel are
    competent in recognition of arrhythmias and evaluation of ischemic symptoms.
    Patients on some forms of vasoactive drips (e.g., low-dose dopamine, dobutamine, or
    nitroglycerin [NTG] infusion) or with a temporary pacemaker already in place may be
    cared for in this unit.

(continued)

Table 3. Definition of unstable angina care environments (continued)

Standard Hospital Unit

A standard hospital unit typically has a nurse to patient ratio greater than 1:5, ECG telemetry may or may not be available, but the nurses must be competent in recognition of unstable angina and its initial management. Access to cardiac resuscitation is via a code cart on the floor and a designated code team. Nursing personnel on the floor are trained in BLS. Continuous heparin infusions may be used, but usually vasoactive drug infusions are not permitted.

411.1) increased from 130,000 in 1983 to 570,000 in 1991 (Graves, 1993; National Center for Health Statistics, 1985). Nearly 60 percent of persons admitted to the hospital with unstable angina as their primary diagnosis were older than age 65, and 46 percent were women. The number of hospitalizations for unstable angina is greater for men than women in all age groups under 75 years of age. The ratio appears to reverse between the ages of 75 and 84, and more women than men are hospitalized for unstable angina over the age of 85 (Feinlieb, Havlik, Gillum

In a further effort to control costs, it is recommended that not every patient admitted with the diagnosis of unstable angina needs to be admitted to an ICU. In fact, the guideline goes to great lengths to define various care environments which may be appropriate for managing patients with unstable angina. The ED and the outpatient clinics hardly need defining. However, the inpatient areas are divided into three types based largely on the nurse to patient ratio and the types of treatment available. Most patients with unstable angina do not need to be admitted to a traditional ICU or CCU with intensive nursing and aggressive treatment and monitoring capabilities, since most are not at high risk. However, the standard hospital unit is not ideal for most unstable angina patients, since there is a small nurse to patient ratio and monitoring and special care are usually not available. Thus, the intermediate care unit or subacute care unit (SAC) is most important for the management of unstable angina patients. Most of these units have an intermediate nurse to patient ratio between an ICU and a standard ward unit and do provide ECG monitoring, the capability for administering IV drugs, and trained personnel competent in ACLS. Clearly, hospitals without such units will be at disadvantage for managing unstable angina patients in a highly cost-effective, yet safe, manner. When we opened a cardiac SAC unit several years ago we found that it immediately reduced ICU/CCU admissions by 50 percent.

Table 4.   Grading of evidence

	Strength of evidence = A	Strength of evidence = B	Strength of evidence = C
Primary evidence	Randomized controlled trials	Well designed clinical studies	Panel consensus
Secondary evidence	Other clinical studies	Clinical studies related to topic but not in an unstable angina population	Clinical studies related to topic but not in an unstable angina population

et al., 1989). This reversal in hospitalizations reflects the larger representation of women than men in advanced age populations and is not due to a change in the relative incidence of CAD diagnosis in men and women in this age group.

Process of Unstable Angina

Precipitating conditions for unstable angina may be those that increase myocardial oxygen demand (e.g., physical exertion) or reduce myocardial oxygen supply (e.g., anemia, development of a platelet-rich thrombus on a fissured plaque, or spasm of an epicardial coronary artery). Unstable angina most often results from disruption of an atherosclerotic plaque and a subsequent cascade of pathologic processes that decrease coronary blood flow (Davies and Thomas, 1984; Falk, 1989; Fuster, Badimon, Badimon et al., 1992; Sherman, Litvack, Grundfest et al., 1986). Most patients who die during unstable angina do so because of sudden death or an intervening MI. Therefore, no pathologic endpoint can be used to define unstable angina.

Unstable angina is often associated with significant angiographic progression of coronary atherosclerotic disease (Moise, Theroux, Taeymans et al., 1984). Patients with unstable angina do have more complex lesions and more coronary thrombus on coronary arteriograms than patients with stable angina (Ahmed, Bittl, and Braunwald, 1993). However, no coronary angiographic findings are pathognomonic of unstable angina. The disorder is often angiographically indistinguishable from non-Q-wave MI (Ambrose, Hjemdahl-Monsen, Borrico et al., 1988; Arbustini, Grasso, Diegoli et al., 1991).

Time-Dependent Mortality Risks of Unstable Angina

Unstable angina presents as a constellation of clinical symptoms and can be legitimately defined in many different ways. The strictness of the definition of unstable angina used and method of assigning deaths to this cause or other ischemic heart disease (IHD) diagnoses can greatly influence reported mortality rates. Moreover, published series of patients with unstable angina commonly begin with

After an extensive literature review, only three types of medical articles were considered by the panel. The most important were randomized clinical trials, which were given a quality rating of A. Second were what were considered excellent clinical studies, which were given a rating of B, and finally, good clinical studies, which were given a rating of C. Each recommendation in the guideline is accompanied by a quality of the scientific evidence grading based on the above letter grades. It is interesting to note how many critical management points made in the guideline are given the rating of C. This is due to the general lack of randomized clinical trials and excellent clinical studies in the area of unstable angina. This makes the consensus opinion of the panel even more important and, like any committee decision, these recommendations always represent a compromise among the various members on the panel. It is stated that the guideline document was field tested for practicality, but few details of the field testing are given and no publications related to this testing have emerged.

Evidence-based medical practice is an attractive concept that has been used to explain the lower rates of revascularization for coronary artery disease in the northeastern United States, as compared to the rest of the United States, but it has limitations. If there is no pertinent literature for a certain clinical problem, then the practitioner of evidence-based medicine runs the risk of doing less than should be done for the patient. It is probably better to be proactive for the patient as long as no harm is done, until subsequent studies show otherwise. All clinical trials select patients based upon entrance criteria that the patient you are treating may not meet. So the trial results do not often help you with your patient. Finally, some management approaches will never be studied for a variety of reasons and we must decide based upon our own experience how to deal with certain patients. If costs are allowed to influence such decisions they will be different than when cost is no object. In my experience the applicability of evidence-based medicine is small in the CAD population.

the definitive diagnosis of the condition and not at the onset of symptoms. Therefore, the mortality observed in any series of carefully defined patients with unstable angina will tend to understate the risk in comparison with the mortality rate expected for these patients at the time of initial presentation for acute chest pain. The diagnosis of unstable angina at the time of hospital admission carries a risk of death that is intermediate between the IHD diagnoses of stable angina and acute MI. This fact is well illustrated by data from the Duke Cardiovascular Databank describing the rate of cardiac death in 21,761 patients treated for CAD without interventional procedures at Duke University Medical Center (DUMC)

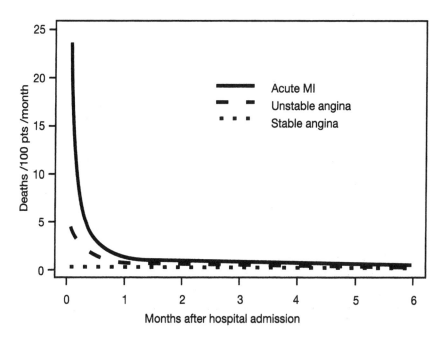

Figure 1.   Outcomes of 21,761 medically treated patients at Duke University Medical Center, 1985–1992, grouped by ischemic heart disease diagnosis on admission.
Source: Unpublished data, Duke Cardiovascular Databank.

between 1985 and 1992 (see Figure 1). The three patient groups were defined by the diagnoses of stable angina, unstable angina, or acute MI at the time of admission. All three groups of patients had the highest risk of cardiac death at the time of presentation, and the risk declined so that by 2 months, mortality rates were indistinguishable in all three populations.

Figure 2 shows the rate of death over time in the same subgroup of 9,146 medically treated patients with an admission diagnosis of unstable angina as in Figure 1 but on an expanded scale. Mortality data from 15 published series (Table 5) are overlaid on the Duke data by straight lines that depict the average mortality (height of the line) over the specific time interval (the beginning and ending of the line). These data demonstrate the mortality of unstable angina to be greatest at time of hospital admission and to rapidly decline over the 2 months thereafter.

Diagnosis of Unstable Angina
In patients without a known history of CAD, consideration of the diagnosis of CAD demands assessment of whether the patient's presentation, with its constellation of specific symptoms and signs, is most consistent with CAD or with an alternative disease process.

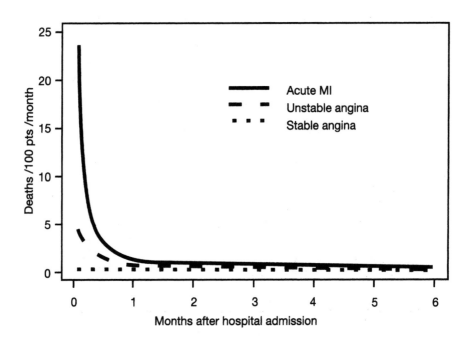

Figure 2. Outcomes of medically treated patients with unstable angina.
Source: Published data as shown in Table 5 and unpublished data, Duke Cardiovascular Databank.

Findings by history useful for establishing the likelihood of CAD.   The five major factors of the initial history and physical examination that relate to the likelihood of CAD are ranked in order of importance (Chaitman, Bourassa, Davis et al., 1981; Pryor, Harrell, Lee et al., 1983; Pryor, Shaw, McCants et al., 1993).

- Angina description by physician (definite angina, probable angina, probably not angina, not angina).
- Prior MI (history, ECG Q-waves).
- Sex.
- Age.
- Number of risk factors (diabetes, smoking, hypercholesterolemia, hypertension).

Character of angina.   Angina is characterized as a deep, poorly localized chest or arm discomfort that is reproducibly associated with physical exertion or emotional stress and relieved promptly by rest or sublingual NTG. Patients with unstable angina may have all the qualities of typical angina except that episodes are more severe and prolonged and may occur at rest with an unknown relation-

Table 5.   Reported mortality of unstable angina

Letter in Figure 2	Primary study	Definition for entry	Patients entered	Study interval	Deaths/100 patients/ month
A	Clinical trial: lidocaine vs. placebo	EMT diagnoses of possible acute MI	1,427	Prehospital, presenting to paramedics	4.2
B	Multicenter Chest Pain Trial	Increasing New onset	3,465	Presenting at ED	2.6
			458	Postdischarge to approximately 2.3 years	1.0
C	Natural history of angina patients	Increasing	4,698	Presenting at ED	5.0
				ICU discharge to 1 year	0.2
D	Clinical trial: aspirin vs. heparin	Increasing ECG changes	484	First 3 days of ICU admission	2.0
E	Clinical trial: nifedipine vs. propranolol plus nitrate	Rest Increasing	133	ICU Admission to 2 weeks	6.0
				2 weeks post-admission to 6 months	0.4
F	Reaction to discontinuing heparin	Increasing New onset ECG changes	403	Day 7–11 of ICU admission	1.6

(continued)

Table 5.   Reported mortality of unstable angina (Continued)

Letter in Figure 2	Primary study	Definition for entry	Patients entered	Study interval	Deaths/100 patients/ month
G	Prognostic significance of ECG	Rest Increasing New onset	911	ICU admission to 1 year	0.2
H	Clinical trial: propranolol vs. diltiazem	Increasing New onset ECG changes	100	Discharge to 1 month post- presentation	4.8
I	Outcome of unstable angina	Rest Increasing	196	Discharge to 4 months	0.75
J	Describe events for ICU patients	Rest Increasing No enzymes	4,698	ICU discharge to 1 year	0.5
K	Smoking outcomes	None	157	Months 2–6 postpresentation	1.0
L	Clinical trial: Enalapril vs. placebo	Ejection fraction	6,797	Screening to average of 40 months	0.5
M	Clinical trial: Antihyper- tensives vs. placebo	Age >60 SB >160 DBP >90	5,736	Screening to average of 4.5 years	0.06

Key = A: Hargarten, Aprahamian, Stueven et al., 1986; B: White, Lee, Cook et al., 1990; C: Karlson, Herlitz, Pettersson et al., 1993; D: Theroux, Waters, Qiu et al., 1993; E: Muller, Turi, Pearle et al., 1984; F: Theroux, Waters, Lam et al., 1992; G: Nyman, Areskog, Areskog et al., 1993; H: Theroux, Taeymans, Morissette et al., 1985; I: Wilcox, Freedman, McCredie et al., 1989; J: Cairns, Singer, Gent et al., 1989; K: Daly, Mulcahy Graham et al., 1983. L: Yusef, Pepine, Garces et al., 1992; M: SHEP Cooperative Research Group, 1991.

ship to exertion or stress. Rest discomfort with all the features of angina but without an exertional component should be considered definite angina for purposes of estimating CAD likelihood. Some patients may have no chest discomfort but present solely with jaw, neck, ear, or arm discomfort. If these symptoms have a clear relationship to exertion or stress or are relieved promptly by NTG, they should be considered equivalent to angina. Occasionally such symptoms at rest may be the mode of presentation of a patient with unstable angina, but without the exertional history, it may be difficult to recognize their cardiac origin. Other difficult presentations of the patient with unstable angina include those without any chest (or equivalent) discomfort. Isolated, unexplained, new onset or worsened exertional dyspnea is the most common such symptom; others include nausea and vomiting and diaphoresis. Assessment of angina should conclude with a summary statement of the patient's symptoms to one of the following four categories: definite angina, probable angina, probably not angina, and not angina (CASS, 1981).

Features suggesting a diagnosis of not angina include:

- Pleuritic pain; i.e., sharp or knife-like pain brought on by respiratory movements or cough.
- Primary or sole location of discomfort in the middle or lower abdominal region.
- Pain localized with one finger.
- Pain reproduced by movement or palpation of chest wall or arms.
- Constant pain lasting for days.
- Very brief episodes of pain lasting a few seconds or less.
- Pain radiating into the lower extremities.

Sharp, stabbing, or pleuritic qualities do not completely exclude an ischemic etiology. In the Multicenter Chest Pain Study, acute ischemia was diagnosed in 22 percent of ED patients presenting with sharp or stabbing pain and 13 percent of patients with some (but not full) pleuritic qualities to the presenting pain. Furthermore, 7 percent of patients whose pain was fully reproduced by palpation were ultimately recognized to have acute IHD (Lee, Cook, Weisberg et al., 1985).

Prior MI, age, gender, and physical findings. Evidence of a prior MI (history or pathologic Q-waves on the resting ECG) or a history of resuscitation from sudden cardiac death indicates a very high likelihood of significant CAD. For any clinical presentation, older patients have a higher CAD likelihood than younger patients, and at any age, men have a higher CAD likelihood than women. The likelihood of CAD and of more severe CAD increases with age, although women who have not undergone premature menopause generally lag 10 years behind men.

Findings on cardiac physical examination of a transient S_3 or S_4 mitral regurgitation murmur or precordial lift during an episode of discomfort signify a high likelihood of significant CAD. The presence of bruits or pulse deficits suggesting extracardiac vascular disease (carotid, aortic, peripheral) identifies patients with a higher likelihood of significant CAD.

Risk factors. Cardiovascular risk factors are modestly predictive of the likelihood of CAD in asymptomatic and nonacute symptomatic patients (Chaitman, Bourassa, Davis et al., 1981; Pryor, Harrell, and Lee, 1983). A clinical diagnosis of diabetes mellitus is the most important risk factor, but cigarette smoking, hypercholesterolemia, and hypertension are also important predictors. A history of premature CAD (age <55) in a parent or sibling has inconsistently been identified as a major risk factor. This association may signify a genetic predisposition to CAD, or reflect the end result of shared environment and lifestyle characteristics, or both.

In the ED, risk factors have been found to be only weakly predictive of the likelihood of acute ischemia in men (diabetes and family history were strongest followed by smoking history); in women, no risk factor was a significant predictor of acute ischemia, possibly due to lower statistical power in this subset. A 50 percent or higher (nonsignificant) increase was seen with diabetes and hypertension (Jayes, Beshansky, D'Agostino et al., 1992). Thus, in patients with suspected unstable angina, risk factors are far less important than the patient's symptoms and ECG findings, and presence or absence of risk factors should not be used to decide whether an individual patient should be admitted or treated for unstable angina.

History of variant angina. Variant angina is an uncommon clinical syndrome of rest pain and reversible ST-segment elevation which may be difficult to diagnose on initial presentation (Table 6). Approximately one-fourth of these patients in the United States have "insignificant" CAD and symptoms due to coronary vasospasm. Thus, this diagnosis may suggest specific management strategies, particularly the use of calcium channel blockers and nitrates and avoidance of beta blockers. However, three-fourths or more of these patients in the United States have a subtotal stenosis in a coronary artery, and a ruptured plaque is often demonstrable when their clinical course becomes unstable (Mark, Califf, Morris et al., 1984; Waters, Miller, Szlachcic et al., 1983). Management of this latter group of patients is similar to that of other patients with unstable angina.

History of cocaine use. Cocaine use has recently been implicated as a cause of unstable angina. Three possible mechanisms by which cocaine induces myocardial ischemia are: (1) increased myocardial oxygen demand (2) decreased myo-

Table 6.   Features suggestive of variant angina

Predominant rest angina
Early morning predominance of attacks
Repetitive chest pain episodes of short duration
Syncope during angina
ST-segment elevation with attacks
Rapid reversibility of ST-elevation
Associated migraine headache or Raynaud's phenomenon

Table 7. ECG findings useful for establishing the likelihood of coronary artery disease

Finding	Most likely cause	Alternate causes
ST-segment elevation ≥1 mm in two or more contiguous leads	Acute MI	Acute pericarditis Early repolarization Left ventricular aneurysm Coronary spasm
ST-segment depression ≥1 mm	Ischemia or acute MI	Normal heart Hyperventilation LV hypertrophy with strain Digitalis Hypokalemia Hypomagnesemia
Inverted T-waves in two or more contiguous leads (≥1 mm in leads with dominant R-waves, or marked symmetrical precordial T-wave inversion)	Ischemia or acute MI	Normal heart Central nervous system disease Hypertrophic cardiomyopathy

cardial oxygen supply secondary to vasospasm or coronary thrombosis, and (3) direct myocardial toxicity. Documented cocaine use should not be considered to rule out underlying significant CAD, since the drug may precipitate coronary vasospasm or acute MI in the patient with atherosclerotic CAD.

ECG Findings Useful for Establishing the Likelihood of CAD. Careful examination of the ECG is crucial in the diagnosis of unstable angina (Rouan, Lee, Cook et al., 1989). A recording made during an episode of the patient's presenting symptoms is particularly valuable, although an asymptomatic recording can be quite informative as well. Importantly, transient ST- or T-wave changes that develop during a symptomatic episode at rest and resolve when the patient becomes asymptomatic strongly suggest unstable angina and a very high likelihood of underlying severe CAD. Patients whose current ECG suggests acute IHD have added diagnostic accuracy if a prior ECG is available for comparison (Lee, Cook, Weisberg et al., 1990). ST-segment and T-wave changes are the primary elements upon which an ECG diagnosis of acute ischemia is based (see Table 7).

ST-segment elevation ≥1 mm in two or more contiguous leads strongly suggests the diagnosis of acute MI and possible candidacy for reperfusion therapy. ST-segment depression typically signifies ischemia or non-Q-wave infarction. Acute reperfusion therapy is usually not indicated for patients with this finding, except for those with acute posterior infarction manifesting the most marked ST-depressions in V_1–V_3. Inverted T-waves may also indicate ischemia or non-Q-wave infarction, especially with T-waves inverted ≥1 mm in leads with dominant

R-waves. Marked symmetrical precordial T-wave inversion strongly suggests acute ischemia, particularly that due to a proximal LAD stenosis. Established Q-waves ≥0.04 seconds are less helpful in the diagnosis of unstable angina, although they do indicate a high likelihood of significant CAD with prior MI. Isolated Q-waves in lead III may be a normal finding.

Nonspecific ST- and T-wave changes, usually defined as ST-deviation or T-wave inversion <1 mm, are less helpful than the foregoing findings. In the Multicenter Chest Pain Study, when such findings were present, approximately one-fourth of the patients had acute IHD (predominantly unstable angina) (Lee, Cook, Weisberg et al., 1985), but this was lower than the prevalence of such disease in the ED population overall. Thus, these nonspecific changes actually lowered the likelihood of MI and unstable angina, but not enough to reliably exclude either diagnosis. In the Multicenter Acute Ischemia Predictive Instrument Trial (Pozen, D'Agostino, Selker et al., 1984), findings were similar. Along with elevation or depression of ST-segments of 1 mm or more, even ST-segment "straightening" (horizontal or downsloping ST-segment with slight depression suggesting acute ischemia) was found to be significantly predictive of the presence of acute ischemia.

A completely normal ECG in the ED does not exclude the possibility of acute IHD, since 1 to 6 percent of such patients will eventually prove to have had an acute MI, and 4 percent or more will be found to have unstable angina (McCarthy, Wong, and Selker, 1990; Rouan, Lee, Cook et al., 1989). In the Multicenter Acute Ischemia Predictive Instrument Trial (Pozen, D'Agostino, Selker et al., 1984), 6 to 7 percent of ED patients with acute ischemia were found to be sent home. In a followup study (McCarthy, Beshansky, D'Agostino, Selker, 1993) that included a search of the National Death Index, it was found that this 6 to 7 percent false-negative discharge rate included 2 percent of ED patients with acute MI who had been sent home. A study by the Multicenter Chest Pain Group showed a 4 percent false-negative discharge rate for acute MI (Rouan, Lee, Cook et al., 1989).

Summary: Estimating the Likelihood of CAD. Clinical and ECG characteristics that relate to the likelihood of significant CAD in groups of patients with symptoms suggestive of unstable angina at the time of initial presentation can be integrated into a summary statement about the likelihood of disease in an individual patient. Estimation of the likelihood of significant CAD is a multivariable problem that cannot be accurately quantitated from a simple table. Therefore, Table 8 is meant only to be illustrative of the general relationships between clinical and ECG findings and three arbitrary groupings of the likelihood of significant CAD. This table may be used to supplement the general clinical impression to categorize an individual patient as having low, intermediate, or high likelihood of CAD.

Determination of Prognosis in Patients with Unstable Angina

Since patients with unstable angina as a group are at increased risk of cardiac death and nonfatal MI, assessment of prognosis often sets the pace of initial eval-

Table 8. Likelihood of significant coronary artery disease in patients with symptoms suggesting unstable angina

High likelihood (e.g., 0.58–0.99)	Intermediate likelihood (e.g., 0.15–0.84)	Low likelihood (e.g., 0.01–0.14)
Any of the following features:	*Absence of high likelihood features and any of the following:*	*Absence of high or intermediate likelihood features but may have:*
History of prior MI or sudden death or other known history of CAD	Definite angina: males <60 or females <70 years of age	Chest pain classified as probably not angina
Definite angina: males ≥60 or females ≥70 years of age	Probable angina: males ≥60 or females ≥70 years of age	One risk factor other than diabetes
Transient hemodynamic or ECG changes during pain	Chest pain probably not angina in patients with diabetes	T-wave flattening or inversion <1 mm in leads with dominant R-waves
Variant angina (pain with reversible ST-segment elevation)	Chest pain probably not angina and two or three risk factors other than diabetes[1]	Normal ECG
ST-segment elevation or depression ≥1 mm	Extracardiac vascular disease	
Marked symmetrical T-wave inversion in multiple precordial leads	ST-depression 0.05 to 1 mm	
	T-wave inversion ≥1 mm in leads with dominant R-waves	

[1]Coronary artery disease risk factors include diabetes, smoking, hypertension, and elevated cholesterol.

Note: Estimation of the likelihood of significant coronary artery disease is a complex, multivariable problem that cannot be fully specified in a table such as this. Therefore, the table is meant to illustrate major relationships rather than offer rigid algorithms.

uation and treatment of patients with suggestive symptoms. For all modes of presentation of IHD, a strong relationship exists between indicators of likelihood of CAD and prognosis. Those patients with a high likelihood of CAD are at a greater risk of an untoward cardiac event than patients with a lower likelihood of CAD. Therefore, assessment of the likelihood of CAD is the beginning point for determining prognosis in a patient presenting with symptoms suggestive of unstable angina. The two other important elements for prognostic assessment are the recent tempo of the patient's clinical course, which relates to the short-term risk of future cardiac events, principally acute MI, and the patient's likelihood of survival should an acute ischemic event occur.

Clinical and ECG Findings Related to Short-Term Prognosis in Patients with Unstable Angina

The tempo of the patient's disease is judged from the cardiac history and ECG and from an examination of the patient during a symptomatic episode. The key elements of the history are: the current frequency of episodes, the change in frequency over the last 2 months (and particularly the last week), any increase in severity or duration of symptoms and in particular occurrence of episodes lasting >20 minutes, progression from effort or stress-related symptoms to symptoms occurring at rest, new onset of nocturnal symptoms, or a significant decrease in the amount of stress or effort necessary to provoke symptoms (Califf, Mark, Harrell et al., 1988; De Servi, Ghios, Ragni et al., 1985). New onset angina is an adverse prognostic event (Roberts, Califf, Harrell et al., 1983), but its risk is defined by other variables from the history, such as the tempo, frequency, and severity of symptoms (Califf, Mark, Harrell et al., 1988; White, Lee, Cook et al., 1990).

Whenever possible, the patient should be examined and have an ECG recorded during a symptomatic episode. The key prognostic elements from the physical examination include any evidence of acute CHF (i.e., new or worsening rales, an S_3), a new or worsening MR murmur, and systemic hypotension. The major prognostic elements from the ECG are dynamic shifts in the ST-segment (≥ 1 mm ST-depression or elevation) or T-wave inversions that resolve, at least partially, when symptoms are relieved (Bosch, Theroux, Pelletier et al., 1991; Karlson, Herlitz, Petterson et al., 1993). With these characteristics it is possible to separate patients into three risk groups as defined in Table 9.

Factors Affecting Both Short- and Long-Term Prognosis in Unstable Angina

The four most important factors related to the likelihood of survival should an acute ischemic event occur in all groups of patients with CAD, including those with unstable angina, are LV function, extent of obstructive coronary artery disease, age, and comorbid conditions. Assessment of LV function is the single strongest predictor of subsequent cardiac death in patients with CAD, and this relates to the lowered reserve of cardiac function in these patients which makes them less tolerant of further ischemia or infarction. The extent of coronary disease defines both the likelihood of an acute coronary event and the likely availability of collateral supply should such an event occur. Thus, coronary events are both more frequent and more likely to be fatal in patients with significant CAD of all three coronary arteries than in patients with significant one-vessel disease. Advanced age is an independent marker of risk that may relate to the lower reserve of cardiac function during stress in the elderly as well as to diminished function of other important organ systems. Important comorbid conditions that greatly influence

Table 9.   Short-term risk of death or nonfatal myocardial infarction in patients with unstable angina

High risk	Intermediate risk	Low risk
At least one of the following features must be present:	*No high-risk feature but must have any of the following:*	*No high- or intermediate-risk feature but may have any of the following features:*
Prolonged ongoing (>20 mins) rest pain	Prolonged (>20 mins) rest angina, now resolved, with moderate or high likelihood of CAD	Increased angina frequency, severity, or duration
Pulmonary edema, most likely related to ischemia	Rest angina (>20 mins or relieved with rest or sublingual nitroglycerin)	Angina provoked at a lower threshold
Angina at rest with dynamic ST changes ≥1 mm	Nocturnal angina	New onset angina with onset 2 weeks to 2 months prior to presentation
Angina with new or worsening MR murmur	Angina with dynamic T-wave changes	Normal or unchanged ECG
Angina with S_3 or new/worsening rales	New onset CCSC[1] III or IV angina in the past 2 weeks with moderate or high likelihood of CAD	
Angina with hypotension	Pathologic Q waves or resting ST depression ≤1 mm in multiple lead groups (anterior, inferior, lateral) Age <65 years	

[1]CCSC = Canadian Cardiovascular Society classification.
Note: Estimation of the short-term risks of death and nonfatal MI in unstable angina is a complex multivariate problem that cannot be fully specified in a table such as this. Therefore, the table is meant to offer general guidance and illustration rather than rigid algorithms.

survival in patients with unstable angina include renal failure, chronic obstructive pulmonary disease (COPD), cerebrovascular disease, and malignancy or other chronic systemic disease.

Computer-Based Risk-Stratification Models in Patients with Acute Ischemic Heart Disease

Based on the disappointing results of using customarily available clinical data, investigators have proceeded to evaluate mathematically-based decision aids and newer cardiac imaging techniques to optimize ED triage of such patients.

The different short-term risk categories delineated in Table 8 also can be conceptualized as representing different points in a spectrum between stable angina at the very low-risk end and acute MI at the very high-risk end. In order of ascending risk, moving from stable angina toward infarction, these categories are: (1) change in anginal threshold (with change of CCSC I to class II or class II to class III being of less concern than a change of class I to class III); (2) accelerating angina (this term indicates a temporally compressed or more recent change in anginal threshold, though no specific criteria are accepted); (3) rest angina or "Angina decubitus" (especially high risk in this category are patients with early morning angina or angina awakening them from sleep); and (4) crescendo angina or "impending infarction" (episodes of increasing severity and duration over the preceding 24 hours) (Hussain et al., 1995B). As previously noted, additional risk applies if episodes are accompanied by ECG changes in the anterior precordial leads or in greater than 4 leads.

Other adverse prognostic factors were recently described in a prospective unstable angina registry study in the Netherlands. (Van Millenburg et al., 1995) They found that resting angina was more important for predicting ongoing ischemia if it had occurred less than 48 hours ago versus greater than 48 hours. Also, infarct-free survival was adversely affected by age and the presence of post-MI angina. Thus, they recommended further subgrouping patients by the timing of rest pain, age, and recent MI. This study also confirmed the importance of ECG changes in predicting risk. An accompanying editorial suggested the following characteristics of a very high risk group (Lindenfeld and Morrison, 1995).

- Rest angina <48 hours
- Post-MI angina
- Reversible ECG changes

The goal of mathematically-based diagnostic aids for acute cardiac ischemia and acute MI is to improve physicians' use of clinical information by quantifying risk in the face of uncertainty (McCarthy, Wong, Selker, 1990; McNutt and Selker, 1988; Wasson, Sox, Neff, Goldman, 1985). The first such diagnostic aid was Sawe's (1972) "clinical diagnostic index," which predicted acute MI based on nine clinical variables derived by discriminant analysis. Tested prospectively it was 100 percent sensitive for acute MI, but its very poor specificity (16%) limited its applicability to actual practice. Based on 655 ED patients with chest pain, Tierney and colleagues created a multivariable model predicting acute MI based on the clinical presentation and ECG that was more specific (86% vs. 78%), but less sensitive (81% vs. 87%) than physicians. Hypothetical integration with physicians' triage decisions did not significantly improve accuracy, and its prospective trial has not been reported (Tierney, Roth, Psaty et al., 1985).

In the Multicenter Chest Pain Study of 12,140 patients, a model was developed using data from the history, physical examination, and ECG to predict the probability of acute MI and improve triage to the ICU (Goldman, Cook, Brand et al., 1988; Goldman, Weinberg, Weisberg et al., 1982). Features associated with a higher probability of acute MI included: duration of symptoms <48 hours prior to ED evaluation, history of angina or prior MI, pain duration ≥1 hour, pain worse than prior angina or equivalent to prior MI, age ≥40, ST- or T-wave changes of ischemia or strain not known to be old, and radiation of pain to the neck, left shoulder, or left arm. Features lowering the probability of acute MI include: radiation of pain to the back, abdomen, or legs; "stabbing" quality of pain; and reproduction of pain by palpation. Combinations of these characteristics yielded 14 subgroups with a probability of acute MI ranging from 1 to 77 percent.

The Multicenter Chest Pain Study model has been shown to stratify 36 percent of patients presenting with chest pain to the ED into a low-risk subgroup (Lee, Juarez, Cook et al., 1991). After a 12-hour observation period, 81 percent of these low-risk subjects remained free of recurrent pain and had at least one normal and no abnormal cardiac enzyme determinations. These uncomplicated low-risk patients were judged to be suitable, after the 12-hour observation period, for further evaluation and therapy in an unmonitored hospital setting. Evidence of acute MI was subsequently obtained in 0.5 percent of this cohort, and 0.6 percent died of cardiac causes during the hospitalization, all after day 3. Further results from this research project showed that initially uncomplicated "rule-out MI" patients can probably be cared for safely in an intermediate care unit, thus reserving ICU admission for patients with definite or high probability for acute MI and patients who have developed early complications (Fiebach, Cook, Lee et al., 1990).

Pozen and colleagues developed and validated a quantitative predictive instrument to improve the diagnosis of acute cardiac ischemia (unstable angina or acute MI) and subsequent triage decisions in the ED (Pozen, D'Agostino, Selker et al., 1984). They identified seven major predictive factors: (1) age; (2) sex; (3) the presence or absence of chest pain or pressure, or left arm pain; (4) whether or not chest pain or pressure was the patient's most important presenting symptom; (5) the presence or absence of ECG Q-waves; (6) the presence and degree of ECG ST-segment elevation and depression; and (7) the presence and degree of ECG T-wave peaking or inversion (Selker, Griffith, and D'Agostino, 1991). This model was shown to have a sensitivity of 95 percent and a specificity of 78 percent for diagnosis of acute cardiac ischemia.

In addition to the use of acute cardiac ischemia as the clinical endpoint instead of acute MI alone, this work is also different from prior work in that instead of only including patients with chest pain, it included all ED patients presenting with symptoms suggestive of acute cardiac ischemia including chest pain or left arm

The bulk of the Overview section describes the background information needed to understand the more detailed management sections that follow. To summarize, it is stated that unstable angina is more common in patients with known CAD and it falls clinically between the spectrum of chronic stable angina and MI. Hence, the majority of patients are greater than age 65 years and about half of unstable angina patients are women, because their incidence of CAD increases in the older age groups. The pathophysiology of unstable angina is in marked contrast to the conservative approach recommended in the guideline. It is well known that patients with unstable angina often have more complex CAD with recent plaque rupture and thrombus formation. This pathophysiology would suggest that an aggressive, invasive approach would be appropriate, but the available literature does not support this contention. The risk of cardiac events or death also lies between the risk of those patients with chronic stable angina and acute MI. Also, the risks decline rapidly after the diagnosis of unstable angina is made and decrease to a level consistent with those with chronic stable angina in about 2 months, regardless of the type of treatment given.

The evaluation of patients with chest pain starts by a classification of their symptom complex into definite angina, probable angina, probably not angina, and not angina. The likelihood that the patient has CAD or the risk of a future event is somewhat related to this classification. Also important is whether there is any other evidence of CAD or vascular disease in the patient. Traditional risk factors are of modest diagnostic value. The presence of diabetes has the best predictive value for coronary disease in patients with chest pain, followed by family history, smoking, and finally, hypertension. Cholesterol elevations tend not to be as useful. Perhaps the most useful clinical tool in the initial evaluation of patients with suspected unstable angina is the ECG. Transient ST- and T-wave changes are highly suggestive of heart disease and Q-waves suggest old MI. However, a normal ECG does not exclude the diagnosis of unstable angina. In fact, 2 to 4 percent of acute MI patients present with a normal ECG.

Based on the clinical evidence and the ECG the physician should determine the likelihood that the patient has CAD. In the guideline, this likelihood is divided into 3 categories: high likelihood, which is an 85 to 99 percent chance of having CAD; low likelihood, which is a 1 to 14 percent chance; and finally, a broad category of intermediate likelihood, which encompasses likelihoods from 15 to 84 percent. Most patients will fall into this intermediate area, fostering the conservative approach suggested by the guideline.

(Continued)

(Continued from previous page)

An intermediate likelihood of CAD includes the following clinical scenarios: definite angina; probable angina in a male >60 years old or a female >70 years old; and probably not angina in a diabetic or a patient with other vascular disease, or in a patient with 2 or 3 other risk factors. ECG changes that categorize a patient as at intermediate risk of CAD include ST-segment depression from 1/2 to 1 mm and any T-wave inversions in leads with dominant R-waves. Consideration of these criteria of categorization supports the concept that most patients will fall into the intermediate likelihood category.

After determining the likelihood of CAD, two other factors are used to assess the prognosis of the patient. First is the tempo of their symptoms, which refers to the rate of acceleration of the symptoms' timing, severity, and any associated symptoms, such as syncope. Second, the physician must consider what the likelihood is that the patient will survive if he or she has an MI. This is determined by the presence of congestive heart failure; mitral regurgitation; hypotension; or transient ECG changes. All of these factors will decrease the likelihood that the patient would survive an MI if it were to occur. It is these 3 factors—the likelihood of CAD, the tempo of the symptoms, and the likelihood of survival for the near future—that determine the prognosis of the patient and the aggressiveness of the diagnostic and therapeutic approach. The panel also suggests that an overall risk can be assigned to the patient based on 3 additional considerations. First, if it is new onset angina of less than 2 weeks duration, the patient is at intermediate risk. If the new onset angina is more than 2 weeks old, the patient is at low risk. If the patient's age is <65 years, he or she is at intermediate risk. If the ECG is normal the patient is at low risk. Finally, the panel suggests that an observation unit in the ED is extremely useful, since low-risk patients can be observed for 12 hours with serial creatinine kinase (CK) assays done. If they are pain-free during this time interval, their CKs are negative, and their ECG does not change, then the probability of a MI or death is less than 1 percent and such patients can be sent home to be evaluated further as outpatients.

Summary:

- Low risk: new onset angina <2 wks, normal ECG
- Intermediate risk: new onset angina <2 wks, age <65 years

pain, abdominal pain or nausea, shortness of breath, and dizziness or lightheadedness. (These inclusion criteria were based in the Imminent MI Rotterdam [IMIR] Study criteria, which have been shown to capture more than 90 percent of all patients in a community with acute cardiac ischemia) (Van der Does, Lubsen, Pool et al., 1976). In controlled prospective trials of the instrument's use, first at Boston City Hospital and then in the Multicenter Predictive Instrument Trial (Pozen, D'Agostino, Selker et al., 1984), it reduced false-positive CCU admissions by 30 percent without an increase in false-negative discharges to home.

The Pozen/Selker model is designed to predict acute cardiac ischemia (acute MI plus unstable angina), while the Goldman model predicts the probability of acute MI. Both were originally developed as tools to improve the cost-effective use of cardiac ICU admissions from the ED. Differences in the models can be attributed to the use of different endpoints, different statistical methodologies, and variability in different clinical data sets. Both models emphasize the importance of prolonged or severe chest pain (or equivalent symptoms), evidence of prior MI, and ST- and T-wave changes on the ECG. Although these predictive statistical models have been prospectively tested in diverse practice settings and hospitals with encouraging results, the panel feels that their routine use in clinical medicine is still some years off. However, practitioners and hospitals should be encouraged to use such an approach as a supplement to the traditional less structured clinical evaluation, if they wish to do so.

2

Guideline: Initial Evaluation and Treatment of Unstable Angina

Commentary by Bruce K. Shively, M.D.

Introduction

Patients with symptoms suggestive of unstable angina present to medical attention either by a telephone call to a medical provider, by a visit to a medical facility, or by emergency transport. The medical provider must appropriately match the intensity and urgency of care with the severity of presenting symptoms. Chapter 1 described the criteria by which clinicians can judge whether a patient's presenting symptoms are consistent with unstable angina and assess the short-term risk of the condition as high, intermediate, or low risk for cardiac events. This chapter describes the initial evaluation and management of patients with unstable angina. Figure 3 depicts the decision logic used to identify patients appropriate to manage using recommendations presented in this guideline.

Objectives of Care

Stabilization of acutely ill patients is the most urgent initial objective. However, for the majority of patients presenting with symptoms suggestive of unstable angina who are obviously stable, triage to the appropriate care environment is the most important early task. A pressing question influencing early care is whether the patient is having an acute MI and has indications for thrombolytic or other reperfusion therapy. During the initial evaluation, until it is clear that high-risk characteristics are not present, it is reasonable to address stabilization and triage of all patients as if they were in a high-risk category.

For all patients, anti-ischemic therapy should be instituted promptly in the ED as soon as a working diagnosis of unstable angina is established. Therapy should

Optimal management of the patient with unstable angina is based on the answers to two distinct questions: what is the probability that the presenting symptoms are due to myocardial ischemia and what is the risk of short-term adverse events if this is so (Figure 3 and Tables 7 and 8). The former issue is resolved by considering the context (risk factors, prior cardiac history) and characteristics of the patient's syndrome (e.g., location of chest discomfort and accompanying symptoms). The latter is assessed primarily by the temporal pattern and severity of symptoms leading up to the encounter with the physician and the presence and type of associated ECG findings. The utility of the distinction between probability of ischemic disease and short-term risk is illustrated by the following examples. In-patient observation of a patient with a syndrome having only a low or intermediate probability of myocardial ischemia may be warranted if the risk of an adverse event is high, as would be the case if the symptoms displayed a crescendo pattern. Conversely, a patient with a history virtually diagnostic of coronary disease will generally not require admission if the symptoms have subsided several days prior to the patient's visit.

As the physician attempts to address the probability of coronary disease and the risk of short-term adverse events, it is advisable to maintain a healthy respect for the uncertainty sometimes inherent in the initial diagnostic effort. ED observation or admission for 12 to 48 hours almost always yields clear answers to these two key questions. A recent study demonstrated that a program designed for evaluating hospitalized patients with chest pain can successfully keep hospital stays at 2 days without increasing complications during a 30-day followup. (Weingarten et al., 1994) This conclusion only applies to patients deemed to be at low risk for complications after admission. Criteria that excluded patients from this analysis included: acute MI; recurrent chest pain on therapy; previous revascularization; planned revascularization; and significant comorbidity. Thus, a low-risk group was identified that could be discharged in an average of 2 days with considerable cost savings.

be directed toward relieving symptoms and stabilizing the patient by preventing ischemic complications, particularly recurrent unstable angina or acute MI.

As the situation permits, the patient should be moved from the ED to the most appropriate environment to monitor complications and minimize psychological stress and cardiac work. However, initial medical therapy in the ED should not be delayed while triage arrangements are made. Patients initially considered to have unstable angina but subsequently found to have an alternate diagnosis should be

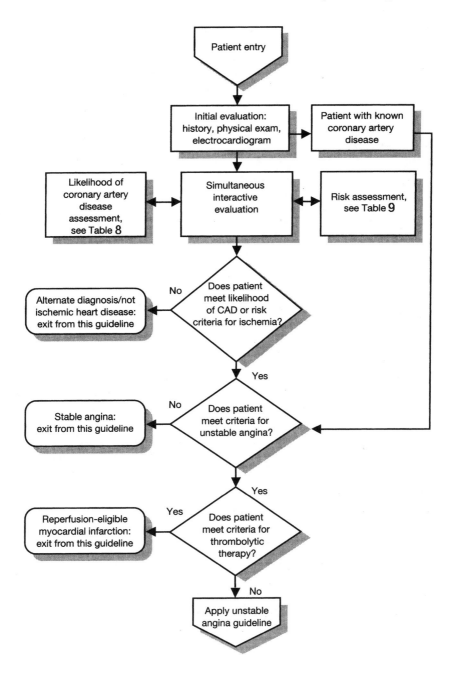

Figure 3. Entry of patients into the unstable angina guideline.

Table 10. Summary of the steps of initial evaluation and treatment

---

Stabilization of vital signs (if necessary).

Initial assessment (brief history of the present illness and ECG). Here the focus is on only the information necessary to place the patient in one of the diagnostic categories on p. 46 of the Guideline: nonischemic symptoms, stable angina, reperfusion eligible myocardial infarction or suspected unstable angina.

Initial treatment (e.g., ASA and heparin).

Detailed assessment (more complete history, including present illness, past cardiac history, and risk factors). After this step the patient should be classified as low-, intermediate-, or high-risk regarding probability of ischemic heart disease and short-term event risk.

Triage (e.g., further observation, admission or home, type of inpatient unit or followup).

Definitive treatment (e.g., additional antianginal drugs, cardiac catheterization).

---

excluded from further management by this guideline at the time the alternate diagnosis is made (see Table 10).

Approach to Care Objectives
Entry into Medical Care Directed by the Guideline
Telephone Presentation.

Recommendation: Because both clinical examination and ECG are critical to early risk assessment, the initial evaluation of the patient with symptoms suggesting possible unstable angina should be done by a medical practitioner in a facility equipped to perform an ECG and not over the telephone (strength of evidence = B).

Health practitioners frequently receive calls from patients who are concerned that the symptoms they notice reflect heart disease. Patients with severe and increasing angina or other symptoms suggesting an impending cardiac catastrophe should be urged to seek transport to an ED. More commonly, telephone calls describe situations that are not clearly urgent, and both the patient and the practitioner often have difficulty knowing which symptoms can be ignored or explored as a nonemergent problem and which should receive more immediate attention.

Patients with known CAD—including those with a recent MI, CABG, or PTCA—who contact their physician because of exacerbation or recurrence of symptoms should, in most instances, be encouraged to seek direct medical care. Only those patients who have been recently evaluated and who are calling for advice regarding modification of medication as part of an ongoing treatment plan represent exceptions to this principle.

Most telephone calls from patients without known CAD regarding chest dis-

The information obtainable by phone is usually insufficient to make it safe to advise the patient not to see a care provider. This stems from the diversity of chest discomfort syndromes and uncertainty in the initial assessment of etiology and short-term risk. It is strongly advised that chest discomfort triage decisions not be made over the phone, despite the potential cost savings in unnecessary ED visits. Any such savings would likely be eliminated by the cost of subsequent morbidity, mortality, and litigation of those with acute ischemic heart disease.

comfort of possible cardiac origin do not represent an emergent situation but simply reflect the desire of the patient for reassurance about the absence of disease or the safety of the symptoms described even if coronary disease might later be found to be present. Despite this fact, nonemergent patients seeking telephone advice for possible cardiac symptoms should be advised that recognition of CAD and evaluation of its severity generally cannot be adequately done by telephone because of the need for an ECG.

The importance of an ECG in early evaluation of unstable angina was emphasized in a study of 90 patients with unstable angina that documented ST-segment deviation >1 mm in two or more leads on ECG to have a positive predictive value for adverse clinical events of 79 percent and a negative predictive value of 64 percent in early evaluation of unstable angina (Cohen, Hawkins, Greenberg et al., 1991). In a study by the Research Group on Instability in CAD in Southeast Sweden (RISC), an abnormal initial ECG was found to be present in 55 percent of 911 men at the time of ICU admission, and ST-segment abnormality was found to be predictive of 76 percent of subsequent death or MI events observed in the population after 90-day followup (Nyman, Areskog, Areskog et al., 1993).

Patients must retain the ultimate responsibility of deciding whether they will seek medical attention and if so in what environment. A medical practitioner cannot be expected to assume responsibility for a patient with a potentially severe cardiac condition who does not present for direct evaluation. Practitioners should be cautious not to provide inappropriate reassurance to patients inclined not to seek further medical attention. However, medical practitioners may assist by providing information patients may use to decide the degree of urgency with which to seek care. The *Patient and Family Guide, Managing Unstable Angina,* is a good source of this information, and this companion booklet, which was developed in conjunction with this guideline, is available free of charge from the AHCPR.

Outpatient Facility or Emergency Presentation.

Recommendation: Patients with suspected unstable angina who have a symptom duration >20 minutes, hemodynamic instability, or recent loss of consciousness should generally be referred to an ED. Other patients with suspected unstable angina may be seen initially either in an ED or in an

> Hypotension and recent loss of consciousness indicate the need for a very aggressive management strategy, but are uncommon. Other more common high-risk features indicating the need to be seen promptly in an ED deserve emphasis. These include, in addition to symptom duration >20 minutes, diaphoresis, severe pain, dyspnea, awareness of a rapid heart beat, and a sense of impending doom. Further, an evaluation in-person is appropriate if the chest discomfort leading the patient to seek medical attention has not been experienced before and is more than mild.

outpatient facility at the discretion of the attending physician (strength of evidence = C).

The decision about where to perform the initial patient evaluation must be based on the individual patient's presenting complaint and circumstances, the options for transportation, and the local facilities available. In general, patients with unremitting symptoms >20 minutes in duration, with symptoms suggesting acute or worsening congestive heart failure (CHF), such as increasing dyspnea or orthopnea, and those with syncope or near-syncope, should be encouraged to go to (or to be transported to) an ED. Transport of these patients by emergency medical transport teams is preferable when readily available. Transport as a passenger in a private vehicle is an acceptable alternative if waiting for an emergency vehicle would impose a long delay. All other patients may be seen initially in an outpatient facility mutually agreeable to the patient and physician.

The first 10 to 20 minutes of the initial encounter with the patient should include a brief assessment of the urgency with which evaluation must be done and treatment started. The urgency of evaluation for patients with ongoing rest pain upon presentation is substantially greater than for patients whose symptoms have already resolved. If the patient is hemodynamically stable and does not appear in great distress, the initial evaluation can precede treatment decisions. Otherwise, both must be done simultaneously. Diagnosis of hemodynamic instability is based on the patient's systolic blood pressure (SBP) (i.e., ≤ 90 mmHg), respiratory status (i.e., acutely dyspneic), mental state (i.e., confused or obtunded), and peripheral circulation (i.e., vasoconstricted, diaphoretic).

No data are available prospectively comparing outcomes of patients treated in different initial care environments and grouped by the severity of presenting cardiac symptoms. Studies of disposition of patient groups after ED presentation for complaints of possible cardiac etiology suggest practitioners must identify the minority of patients with potentially severe disease from within the much larger group of patients who either have no CAD or at least no need for urgent care. In one study of more than 12,140 patients presenting to EDs of three university and

It would be a mistake to infer that information such as this is useful for establishing an a priori probability of coronary disease and guiding initial management. The characteristics of patient populations in different communities or health plans may differ markedly with regard to CAD risk. For example, in a Department of Veterans Affairs hospital or a managed care plan serving mainly senior citizens the percentage of noncardiac chest pain may be 10 percent or less. "Guilty until proven innocent" (of having an ischemic etiology) is an appropriate philosophy.

four community hospitals for evaluation requiring consideration of acute IHD, noncardiac chest pain was diagnosed in about 65 percent (White, Lee, Cook et al., 1990).

Even in the most urgent subgroup of patients presenting with acute-onset cardiac disorders, time is usually adequate to transport patients to an environment where they can undergo evaluation and treatment (Ghali, Cooper, Kowatly et al., 1993; Schroeder, Lamb, and Hu, 1977). A large study of consecutive patients transported to the ED by ambulance for chest pain suspected to be of cardiac etiology resulted in a final diagnosis of acute MI in about one-third, unstable angina in one-third, and noncardiac etiology in most of the remaining third of this population. Only 1.5 percent of these patients developed cardiopulmonary arrest in the prehospital or ED settings (Hargarten, Chapman, Stueven et al., 1990). These data suggest that patients with acute chest pain are better served by transport to an adequate ED than by compromising the quality of the care environment in an attempt to shorten the initial transport time.

Stabilization and Initial Evaluation

Initial Evaluation of Low- and Intermediate-Risk Patients. Intermediate- and low-risk patients (see Table 9) who arrive at a medical facility in a pain-free state, have unchanged or normal ECGs, and are hemodynamically stable represent more of a diagnostic than an urgent therapeutic challenge. Evaluation begins in these patients by obtaining information from history, physical examination, and ECG to be used to confirm the diagnosis of unstable angina as discussed in Chapter 1. After this initial evaluation, those patients assigned to the definitely not angina category are excluded from further management by this guideline. These excluded patients should be evaluated further for another cause of their symptoms or reassured that their symptoms are likely to be self-limited if a nonthreatening cause has been identified (e.g., anxiety, musculoskeletal pain). Reassurance should be balanced with instructions to return for further evaluation if symptoms worsen or fail to respond to symptomatic medical treatment.

Patients meeting criteria for unstable angina should receive ASA therapy, 160 to 324 mg, as described below, unless contraindications are present. Patients without pain but with definite ischemic ECG changes should be treated during this initial phase as if they have ongoing pain. Patients without ongoing pain or ischemic ECG changes should be further risk-stratified. About one-half of these patients will be known to have CAD for which they have received prior treatment. Management decisions for these patients with known CAD are similar to those for patients without known CAD but with a high likelihood of having CAD.

Details of past medical care most likely to impact on current management decisions include prior assessments of LV function and coronary anatomy, prior revascularization procedures, and recent medication history. The current historic information of greatest importance in these patients is their assessment of the severity and tempo of their symptoms in the context of their prior history. Patients who feel that their symptoms are similar to those experienced during a prior major cardiac event and patients who have undergone coronary angioplasty or a bypass operation within the past year and have intermediate- or high-risk features deserve hospital admission for more thorough evaluation in most cases. Patients with known LV dysfunction or CHF represent another group that should usually be admitted to the hospital. Patients who are at or near maximal medical treatment and who have been symptomatic over the preceding 24 hours deserve hospital admission. Others who should be admitted include patients with a symptom duration ≥1 hour (even without ECG changes), patients with a history of rest pain lasting >20 minutes within the past week, or patients with a two-class worsening of angina (Goldman, Cook, Brand et al., 1988). All low-risk patients with known CAD usually can be managed as described in Chapter 3. Hospitalization may be reasonable in some low-risk patients with known CAD, such as those with other diseases that might confound outpatient management and patients who live in areas remote from an appropriate health care facility.

Patients without known CAD and a high likelihood of CAD are managed ini-

> The critical decision in the initial evaluation is whether or not to send the patient home. Patients should not be sent home unless the short-term adverse-event risk is low, irrespective of the clinicians' estimate of the probability of coronary disease. Brief observation (12 to 48 hours) with ASA and heparin is a relatively inexpensive and wise precaution in borderline situations. Unfortunately, observation beyond 23 hours usually requires hospital admission and many ED observation units are not staffed for IV heparin administration. Thus, in practical terms, the physicians' options are limited by the hospital's capabilities and it is inadvisable for the physician to assume additional litigation risk by compromising patient care to save the health care system money.

tially as if they have high-risk unstable angina. For all other patients without known CAD, the pattern of recent symptoms defines the urgency with which further evaluation should proceed to determine the likelihood of CAD as a cause of symptoms. Patients with an intermediate likelihood of CAD for whom another cause of current symptoms cannot be determined who also appear to be at intermediate risk are usually best managed by hospitalization in a standard or intermediate care bed. Patients with an intermediate likelihood of CAD but low risk deserve further evaluation for the cause of their symptoms. In some cases, it will be logistically reasonable to proceed with a more definitive evaluation in the ED. Alternatively, patients who have been asymptomatic for >24 hours can reasonably be referred to an outpatient facility for definitive workup. However, in most situations, this evaluation should be completed within 72 hours, and patients should always be advised to return to the ED immediately for re-evaluation if symptoms recur, worsen, or fail to respond to prescribed symptomatic therapy. A trial of sublingual NTG may provide useful diagnostic information in some of these patients. All patients should be instructed to observe and later report the influence of medication and activity on symptoms experienced during the interval prior to more definitive evaluation.

Patients with a low likelihood of CAD, especially those with a history of intermediate-risk features who currently do not have ongoing pain, ECG change, or hemodynamic instability, should be evaluated carefully for other causes of the presentation including: musculoskeletal chest pain; gastrointestinal (GI) disorders, such as gastritis, peptic ulcer disease, or cholecystitis; intrathoracic disease, such as esophageal spasm, pneumonia, pleurisy, pneumothorax, or pericarditis; neuropsychiatric disease, such as hyperventilation; or panic disorder. Patients who are found to have evidence of one of these alternative diagnoses should be excluded from management by this guideline and referred appropriately for follow up care. Stable angina may also be diagnosed in this setting, and patients with this diagnosis are excluded from further management by this guideline. Patients for whom a specific diagnosis cannot be made on the brief initial examination should undergo a more definitive evaluation. This evaluation may proceed in the ED or outpatient facility if time permits. Occasionally, admission to a standard hospital unit is required for definitive evaluation of patients with complex presentations.

Definitive evaluation of patients with a low likelihood of CAD and low risk is less urgent than it is for patients at higher risk. If time is not adequate in the ED setting to evaluate these low-risk patients sufficiently to arrive at an alternate diagnosis or to differentiate unstable angina from stable angina, patients should be referred for outpatient evaluation, generally within 72 hours, as described in Chapter 3 (see Table 11).

Evaluation of Unstable Angina Patients for Precipitating Noncardiac Causes of Symptoms.

Recommendation: The definitive initial evaluation of the unstable angina patient should include a systematic search for precipitating noncardiac causes

Table 11.   Who should be admitted?

High risk of an event	All
Intermediate and low risk	Known LV dysfunction
	On near-maximal medical therapy
	High likelihood or known CAD
	Intermediate likelihood plus intermediate risk
	Rest angina for >20 minutes
	Two-class worsening of angina
	Significant comorbidities
	Geographic isolation

that might explain the new development of unstable symptoms or the conversion from a stable to an unstable course. Thus, each patient's ECG should be evaluated for arrhythmias, and patients should have a measurement of body temperature and blood pressure, a hemoglobin or hematocrit determination, and a physical examination for evidence of other cardiac diseases (particularly aortic valve disease and hypertrophic cardiomyopathy) or hyperthyroidism (exophthalmos, resting tremor, thyroid exam). Review of the history may reveal additional potential exacerbating factors such as a recent increase in physical activity level especially in combination with environmental temperature extremes, noncompliance with medical therapy, or a recent increase in psychological stress levels (strength of evidence = C).

Information from the initial history, physical examination, and ECG will enable the practitioner to recognize and exclude patients classified as not angina. The remaining patients should undergo more complete evaluation for secondary causes of the presentation and for manifestations of coexisting diseases that might alter management. Cardiac disorders other than CAD that may present with acute ischemia, particularly in the setting of significant CAD, include aortic stenosis and hypertrophic cardiomyopathy. Factors that increase the oxygen demand or decrease myocardial oxygen delivery to the heart may provoke or exacerbate ischemia, particularly in the presence of significant CAD. Previously unrecognized gastrointestinal bleeding is one common secondary cause of exacerbated CAD symptoms due to anemia. Acute worsening of chronic obstructive lung disease (with or without superimposed infection) may lower oxygen saturation levels enough to worsen CAD symptoms. Evidence of increased cardiac oxygen demand over normal resting levels can be judged from the presence of a fever or findings of hyperthyroidism. Similarly, uncontrolled hypertension can increase oxygen demand by making the heart work harder to eject blood during each systole (increased afterload). Sustained supraventricular or ventricular tachycardias may also provoke acute ischemic symptoms (see Table 12).

Table 12.   Precipitating or noncoronary causes of unstable angina (secondary unstable angina)

Arrhythmias	Sinus tachycardia
	Supraventricular tachycardia
	Ventricular tachycardia
Infections	Fever
	Sepsis
High output states	Thyrotoxicosis
	Sympathicominetics
	Hyperadrenergic state (psychologic stress)
Hemodynamic factors	Aortic stenosis
	Hypertrophic cardiomyopathy with obstruction
	Severe systemic hypertension
	Severe congestive heart failure
Reduced oxygen delivery	Anemia
	Hypoxia
	CO poisoning

Initial Evaluation of High-Risk Patients.

Recommendation: The initial assessment of the high-risk patient with possible unstable angina must start with a rapid evaluation of the probability of immediate adverse outcomes and the need for emergency diagnostic and therapeutic interventions. Patients with ongoing symptoms, hemodynamic instability, or recent loss of consciousness should have a directed history, physical examination, and 12-lead ECG completed within 20 minutes of arrival to a medical facility (strength of evidence = B). Specific diagnoses that must be explicitly considered are acute MI meeting criteria for reperfusion therapy, aortic dissection, leaking or ruptured thoracic aneurysm, pericarditis with tamponade, pneumothorax, and pulmonary embolism. Other non-cardiovascular diagnoses may need to be considered as well, depending on initial findings (strength of evidence = B).

Patients who have ongoing symptoms of unstable angina at rest when first seen deserve more urgent evaluation than patients with prior discomfort who are asymptomatic when first seen. Intensive medical treatment, as described in Chapter 4, should begin immediately in the ED in patients with ongoing rest pain or definite ECG ischemia and should continue as the patient is transported to the definitive care environment. Ongoing rest pain with treatment should drive initial evaluation at a more urgent pace and therapy to more aggressive regimens than is required for patients with pain that resolves rapidly as treatment is begun.

Occasionally, patients with rest angina also have hemodynamic instability

Although it is true that the presence of continuing chest discomfort often identifies a high-risk patient, it should be emphasized that this is not the only high-risk identifier. One of the most important high-risk features is the presence of unequivocal new ECG ST-segment shifts or T-wave inversion. The highest risk patients in this or any group with ECG changes are those with changes localized to the anterior precordial leads (indicating a culprit lesion in the anterior descending coronary artery); within this group, the highest risk patients of all are those with changes in leads V_1 and V_2, indicating a proximal anterior descending lesion. Involvement of multiple leads (>4) also implies additional risk. Other ECG features indicating high short-term risk are tall T-waves and QTc prolongation, primarily if new and accompanied by chest discomfort. Other ECG changes indicating short-term risk include newly horizontal ST-segments (i.e., if previously normal with upsloping morphology), T-wave flattening, diffuse ST-T abnormality of uncertain age and perhaps U-wave inversion. (Salahas et al., 1995; Hussain et al., 1995; Arijseels et al., 1995).

manifested by hypotension, dyspnea, and/or a sense of impending catastrophe. Patients who appear unstable should have simultaneous evaluation and treatment. IV access can be obtained while a brief cardiovascular history and physical examination are completed and an ECG is taken. When initial blood work is obtained, a sample should be sent for determination of creatinine kinase (CK). Medical personnel trained in cardiopulmonary resuscitation should remain in close attendance during the period of initial stabilization. Oxygen should be administered by mask or nasal cannula.

A record review of 445 patients presenting to 10 metropolitan EDs for management of acute nontraumatic chest pain found 78 percent of patients underwent physician evaluation and 60 percent had an initial ECG within 20 minutes of arrival in the ED (Heston and Lewis, 1992). This unselected population included patients presenting with a spectrum of severity. It is, therefore, reasonable that all patients presenting with severe symptoms be evaluated for risk within 20 minutes of arrival at the ED. In ED environments without a physician continuously present, nurses or other medical providers should assess the patient, obtain an ECG, and begin treatment to support any patient with hemodynamic instability and involve the physician in important decisions using telecommunications as appropriate to the specific circumstances occurring before the arrival of the physician in the ED.

As treatment is begun in patients with the presumptive diagnosis of high-risk unstable angina, further evaluation should continue to address other possible conditions as alternate diagnoses to unstable angina. Other severe conditions to be considered include acute MI, aortic dissection, leaking or ruptured thoracic

Table 13.   Features of very high risk patients in whom immediate cardiac catheterization is usually indicated

---

A history of left main or proximal LAD stenosis or prior angioplasty or ECG changes suggesting ischemia in this distribution.

A history of recent (<2 weeks) hospital discharge following acute MI.

ECG showing reversible ST-segment elevation, ST- or T-wave changes in leads V1–V4 or in >4 leads.

Recurrent symptoms in the ED or shortly after admission, especially if after receiving ASA or heparin.

Symptoms unrelieved in the ED (20 minutes is a reasonable but rough rule of thumb).

---

aneurysm, acute pericarditis with tamponade, pulmonary embolism, pneumothorax, esophageal rupture, or rupture or ischemia of intra-abdominal organs. Chest or abdominal images (chest radiograph, transthoracic or transesophageal echocardiogram, computed tomogram, or magnetic resonance image) may be useful for differentiating these severe conditions from unstable angina at this early stage of evaluation. However, a history and physical examination directed by suspicion of one of these conditions remains the most important diagnostic tool. In one study of 918 consecutive patients evaluated for suspicion of unstable angina, common alternate final diagnoses included unspecified chest pain, pulmonary embolism, acute abdominal disease, and other miscellaneous diseases (Aase, Jonsbu, Liestol et al., 1993) (see Table 13).

Initial Treatment of Patients with Unstable Angina
Initial General Care.

Recommendation: Patients with unstable angina and ongoing rest pain

> Cardiac catheterization is essential for prompt and accurate risk-stratification of these patients, and in most cases percutaneous or surgical revascularization will probably be indicated (Mureyra et al., 1995). The rapid and definitive diagnosis and treatment implied by this strategy are not necessarily more costly due to savings in hospital days as well as reduction of short- and long-term complications. If the indication for immediate catheterization is recognized early enough, heparin should not be given prior to transfer to the laboratory; it will be given later once vascular access is obtained. Infrequently, cases are encountered in which the potential for immediate discharge of the patient and avoidance of subsequent unnecessary ED visits can be realized by cardiac catheterization direct from the ED if the angiogram shows no significant coronary artery stenoses.

should be placed at bed rest during the initial phase of medical stabilization (strength of evidence = C).

Recommendation: Patients with obvious cyanosis, respiratory distress, or high-risk features (see Table 9) should receive supplemental oxygen. A finger pulse oximetry or arterial blood gas determination should be used to confirm adequate arterial oxygen saturation and continued need for supplemental oxygen (strength of evidence = C).

Recommendation: As soon as the diagnosis of unstable angina is made, patients should be placed on continuous ECG monitoring for ischemia and arrhythmia detection (strength of evidence = C).

The severity of symptoms of unstable angina will dictate some of the general patient care that should be employed during initial treatment of patients with a diagnosis of unstable angina. Patients should be placed on bed rest while ischemia is ongoing but can be mobilized to a chair and bedside commode once they become symptom-free. Subsequent activity restriction should be focused on preventing recurrent symptoms and may be liberalized as judged appropriate as patients respond to treatment. Patients with cyanosis, respiratory distress, or high-risk features (see Table 9) should receive supplemental oxygen, and adequate blood arterial saturation should be confirmed by direct measurement or pulse oximetry. No evidence is available to support the common medical practice of administering oxygen to all patients with acute chest pain syndromes in the absence of signs of respiratory distress. Although routine use of oxygen during initial evaluation would not appear to cause much harm, more selective use of oxygen for patients with questionable respiratory status or those with documented hypoxemia by finger pulse oximeter is a preferable strategy. All patients with unstable angina should undergo cardiac monitoring during their ED evaluation.

Initial Pharmacologic Treatment.[1]   Drugs to be considered for use at the time of initial evaluation and treatment of patients with symptoms suggestive of unstable angina include ASA, heparin, nitrates, and beta blockers. The certainty of diagnosis, severity of symptoms, hemodynamic state, and medication history will determine the choice and timing of drugs used in individual patients. Treatment with an indicated drug should begin in the ED and not be delayed until hospital admission. The aggressiveness of drug dosage will depend on the severity of symptoms and, for many drugs, will require modification throughout the subsequent hospital course. Principles of drug use are not altered by the care environment in which the drug is administered.

---

[1]Some of the recommendations in this guideline suggest the use of agents for purposes or in doses other than those specified by the Food and Drug Administration (FDA). Such recommendations are made after consideration of concerns regarding nonapproved indications. Where made, such recommendations are based on more recent clinical trials or expert consensus.

Table 14. Summary of drugs commonly used in the emergency department to treat patients with symptoms suggestive of unstable angina

Drug category	Clinical condition	When to avoid[1]	Usual dose (low-high)
Aspirin	Diagnosis of unstable angina or acute MI	Hypersensitivity, active bleeding, severe bleeding risk	324 mg (160–324)
Heparin	Unstable angina in high-risk category and some inter-mediate-risk patients	Active bleeding, history of heparin-induced throm-bocytopenia, severe bleeding risk, recent stroke	80 units/kg IV bolus with constant IV infusion at 18 units/kg/hr titrated to maintain aPTT between 46 and 70 seconds2
Nitrates	Ongoing pain or ischemia	Hypotension	Sublingual (1–3 tablets)3 IV (5–100 m g/min)
Beta blockers	Diagnosis of unstable angina	PR ECG segment <0.24 seconds, 2° or 3° AV block, heart rate >60, systolic blood pressure >90 mmHg, shock, left ventricular failure with CHF, severe reactive airway disease	Oral dose appropriate for specific drug IV metoprolol (1–5 mg slow IV every 5 minutes to 15 mg total) IV propranolol 0.5 to 1.0 mg IV atenolol 5 mg every 5 minutes to 10 mg total

(continued)

To avoid redundancy, a detailed description of the use of each drug will be presented only once in this guideline, although modifications of drug use required during other phases of care will be mentioned when appropriate. Because ASA and heparin are the drugs that should be considered early in the treatment of unstable angina, their use is described in this chapter. Nitrates, beta blockers and narcotics are often begun in the ED, but their use at maximum dosage and the importance of response to these agents for determining the need for alternate therapies in individual patients often occurs in the intensive care environment. For this reason the use of nitrates, beta blockers, and morphine is discussed in detail in Chapter 4. Table 14 summarizes indications, contraindications, and usual dosage of drugs commonly used in the ED to treat patients with unstable angina.

Table 14.   Summary of drugs commonly used in the emergency department to treat patients with symptoms suggestive of unstable angina (Continued)

Drug category	Clinical condition	When to avoid[1]	Usual dose (low-high)
Narcotics	Persistent pain following initial therapy with nitrates and beta blockers	Hypotension, respiratory depression, confusion, obtundation	Morphine sulfate 2 to 5 mg IV

[1]Allergy or prior intolerance contraindication for all.

[2]Dose regimen assumes a mean control aPTT of 30 seconds and a therapeutic goal of 1.5 to 2.5 times control..

[3]Patients with symptoms suggestive of unstable angina and ongoing pain should be given sublingual NTG 0.3 to 0.4 every 5 minutes until discomfort is relieved, three tablets have been given, or limiting symptoms or signs develop. If discomfort is still present after three tablets, IV NTG should be started promptly at a dose of 5 $gmg/min and titrated up to 75 to 100 $gmg/min or limiting side effects.

Note: Some of the recommendations in this guideline suggest the use of agents for purposes or in doses other than those specified by the Food and Drug Administration (FDA). Such recommendations are made after consideration of concerns regarding nonapproved indications. Where made, such recommendations are based on more recent clinical trials or expert consensus.

Recommendation: IV thrombolytic therapy is not indicated in patients who do not have evidence of acute ST-segment elevation or left bundle branch block (LBBB) on their 12-lead ECG (strength of evidence = A).

The failure of IV thrombolytic therapy to improve clinical outcomes in the absence of acute MI with ST-segment elevation or LBBB has now been clearly demonstrated (TIMI IIIA, 1993; TIMI IIIB, 1994). A meta-analysis by Duke University staff of recent studies of thrombolytic therapy in unstable angina patients shows no benefit of thrombolysis versus standard therapy for the reduction of acute MI. Thrombolytic agents had no significant effect and actually increased the risk of MI by 1.7 percent (95 percent confidence interval [CI] 2.4–5.8%) (Figure 4). Consequently, such therapy is not recommended for unstable angina patients managed according to this guideline.

The distinction between unstable angina and acute MI often cannot be definitively made during the initial evaluation. Patients with ECG changes diagnostic of epicardial injury (i.e., ≥ 1 mm ST-elevation in two or more contiguous leads, or ST-depression in V_1–V_3) or LBBB with a consistent history should be managed as if they have an acute MI, including prompt administration of ASA, beta blockers, and reperfusion therapy. In most large trials of reperfusion therapy, such patients have a ≥ 95 percent prevalence of acute MI. In the Multicenter Chest Pain Study,

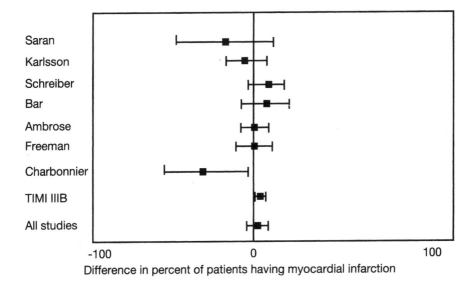

Figure 4.   Influence of thrombolysis on myocardial infarction in patients presenting with unstable angina.
Source: Saran, Bhandari, Narain et al., 1990; Karlsson Berglund, Bjorkholm et al., 1992; Screiber, Rizik, White et al., 1992; Bar, Verheught, Col et al., 1992; Ambrose, Torre, Sharma et al., 1992; Freeman, Langer, Wilson et al., 1992; Charbonnier, Bernadet, Schiele et al., 1992; TIMI IIIB, 1994.

however, only about 80 percent of patients meeting these criteria had acute MI (Lee, Weisberg, Brand et al., 1989).

Recommendation: All patients with the diagnosis of unstable angina should receive regular ASA 160 to 324 mg as soon as possible after presentation unless a definite contraindication is present, such as evidence of ongoing major or life-threatening hemorrhage, a significant predisposition to such hemorrhage (e.g., recent bleeding peptic ulcer disease), or a clear history of severe hypersensitivity to ASA (strength of evidence = A).

The recommendation for an initial ASA to be given in the ED is based on the efficacy of this therapy in independently reducing mortality in patients with acute MI enrolled in the second International Study of Infarct Survival (ISIS-2) trial (1988). Those data, combined with the recognition that a definitive distinction between acute MI and unstable angina is frequently not possible at the time of acute presentation, led to the recommendation to initiate ASA immediately in appropriate patients. No randomized trials or other studies compare immediate with a more delayed initiation of ASA in unstable angina.

Some of the strongest evidence available about the long-term prognostic effects of medical therapy on coronary disease outcomes pertains to ASA. ASA inhibits the formation of thromboxane A_2, thereby diminishing platelet aggregation promoted by some but not all physiologic stimuli. Since platelets are one of the main participants in the thrombotic consequences of disruption of a coronary plaque, platelet inhibition is a plausible mechanism for clinical benefit. In unstable angina, ASA has been shown to have significant benefit for stabilizing an acutely unstable coronary plaque, producing reductions in mortality and MI rates of 50 percent or more.

Four randomized trials clearly demonstrated the benefit of ASA in the long-term treatment of unstable angina. The Veterans Administration (VA) Cooperative Study Group in 1983 compared the effects of 324 mg of ASA given once a day for 12 weeks with the effects of placebo in 1,266 male veterans admitted with unstable angina (Lewis, Davis, Archibald et al., 1983). At the conclusion of the 12-week study period, there was a 51 percent reduction in the rate of nonfatal acute MI in the ASA group (3.4% vs. 6.9%, p = 0.005) and a 51 percent reduction in the rate of death or acute MI in the ASA group (5% vs. 10.1%, p = 0.0005). Although the difference in the mortality rates of the ASA and placebo groups was not significant at 12 weeks, there was a significant 43 percent reduction in the mortality rate of the ASA-treated group at 1-year followup (5.5% vs. 9.6%, p = 0.008).

A group of Swedish investigators reported the effects of ASA (75 mg/day) compared with the effects of placebo in 796 men admitted with either unstable angina or non-Q-wave MI (Wallentin, 1991). Study treatment had been scheduled for 1 year, but the trial was stopped after publication of the ISIS-2 trial. All patients received at least 3 months of treatment. At 12-month followup, there was a significant 48 percent reduction in the combined rate of death and MI in the ASA group (11% vs. 21%, p <0.0001). However, there was no significant difference in the risk of death alone (2.7% vs. 4.5%, p = NS). ASA also reduced the incidence of recurrent angina in this trial.

A Canadian multicenter trial reported in 1985 tested the effects of 325 mg of ASA given every 6 hours with the effects of placebo in 555 patients admitted to the CCU with unstable angina (Cairns, Gent, Singer et al., 1985). At an average followup point of 18 months, there was a significant 56 percent reduction in the risk of cardiac death (5% vs. 9.4%, p = 0.009), although there was no difference in the followup rate of MI. A second Canadian study reported in 1988 examined the effects of 325 mg of ASA given twice per day versus those of placebo in 479 patients admitted to the CCU with unstable angina (Theroux, Ouimet, McCans et al., 1988). The researchers reported a 28 percent reduction in the rate of MI over the first week of therapy in the ASA group (3.3% vs. 11.9%, p = 0.012). There were too few deaths to analyze the effects of the treatment on this endpoint. Meta-analysis of these four studies to assess outcomes measured at greater than 3 months suggests that ASA reduces the risk of MI by 48 percent and the risk of death by 51 percent. There was a 47 percent reduction in the combined risk of death and MI as illustrated in the likelihood function in Figure 5.

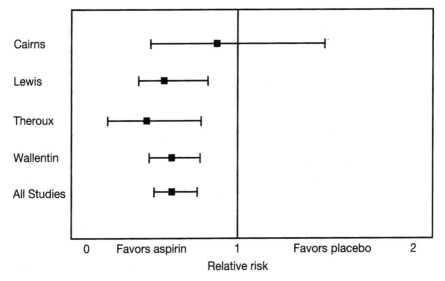

Figure 5.   Relative risk of death or myocardial infarction in unstable angina patients treated with aspirin vs. placebo.
Source: Cairns, Gent, Singer et al., 1985; Lewis, Davis, Archibald et al., 1983; Theroux, Ouimet, McCans et al., 1988; Wallentin, 1991.

No data directly compare the efficacy of different doses of ASA in patients presenting with unstable angina. However, a broad review and meta-analysis of different doses of ASA in long-term treatment of patients with CAD suggest equal efficacy of daily doses of 75 to 324 mg per day (Antiplatelet Trialists' Collaboration, 1994). It appears reasonable to initiate ASA treatment in patients with unstable angina with a dose of at least 160 mg as used in the ISIS-2 (1988) trial. Thereafter, an ASA dose of 80 to 324 mg could be used for long-term therapy.

Recommendation: IV heparin should be started as soon as a diagnosis of intermediate- or high-risk unstable angina is made (strength of evidence = A). The initial dose is 80 units/kg by IV bolus followed by a constant infusion of 18 units/kg/hr, maintaining the activated partial thromboplastin time (aPTT) at 1.5 to 2.5 times control.

There is clear and compelling evidence that IV heparin started early in the course of unstable angina reduces the risk of subsequent MI and recurrent unstable angina. Heparin exerts its anticoagulant effect by markedly accelerating the action of circulating antithrombin III, a proteolytic enzyme that inhibits thrombin and several other activated factors in the clotting cascade. Thus, heparin acts to prevent thrombus propagation but does not lyse existing thrombi (Hirsh, 1991).

Five randomized trials of heparin use in unstable angina have been reported.

Two early trials showed a benefit but must be judged inconclusive due to methodologic defects (Telford and Wilson, 1981; Williams, Kirby, McPherson et al., 1986). A group of Swedish investigators performed a double-blind placebo-controlled trial with a 2 × 2 factorial design in 796 men with unstable angina or non-Q-wave infarction (RISC Group, 1990). The active drug regimens tested were ASA 75 mg daily for ≥3 months and heparin 5,000 units IV bolus every 4 hours. Drug therapy was initiated 1 to 3 days after hospital admission. This investigation did not demonstrate any therapeutic benefit of heparin alone, although patients treated with heparin and ASA combined had significantly fewer (p = 0.0007) deaths and MIs than those treated with heparin alone, and fewer, but not significantly fewer, cardiac events than ASA alone (RISC Group, 1990).

Two placebo-controlled heparin and ASA trials were performed at the Montreal Heart Institute. A 479-patient study performed between 1986 and 1988 tested treatments consisting of 650 mg of ASA immediately followed by 324 mg twice per day and a 5,000-unit IV heparin bolus followed by 1,000 units per hour in a 2 × 2 factorial design (Theroux, Ouimet, McCans et al., 1988). Importantly, a double-blind placebo was used for both heparin and ASA ensuring truly unbiased assessment of efficacy. Although the study was too small to detect an effect on mortality, the risk of MI was reduced by 89 percent and the risk of recurrent refractory angina by 63 percent relative to placebo. In this study, ASA also reduced the rate of MI, but the two drugs given together were not superior to heparin alone (possibly due to the relatively small sample size and inadequate statistical power) and were associated with a slightly higher risk of serious bleeding. A more recent double-blind randomized trial from this group compared ASA (325 mg twice per day) and heparin (5,000 units IV bolus followed by a constant infusion titrated to an aPTT 1.5 to 2.5 × control) in 484 unstable angina patients. MI (fatal or nonfatal) occurred in 0.8 percent of heparin patients and 3.7 percent of ASA patients (p = 0.035). This trial was the first to clearly demonstrate the superiority of IV heparin over ASA in the acute phase of unstable angina (Theroux, Waters, Qiu et al, 1993).

Taken together, these available trials indicate a substantial reduction in acute MI incidence from early heparin, with possible reduction of death and recurrent unstable angina. No direct data exist about the relative efficacy of bolus administration versus continuous infusion of heparin, but two randomized trials from another area of medicine suggest equivalent anticoagulant results and more bleeding complications with intermittent therapy. Thus, although continuous infusion is preferred in this guideline, centers not equipped to administer heparin by continuous infusion may substitute a regimen of 5,000 units IV bolus every 4 hours.

The efficacy of ASA and heparin in combination is suggested, but this benefit has not been unequivocally demonstrated relative to monotherapy by their complementary mechanisms of action and demonstrated value in different phases of the disease. ASA has been shown to provide benefits with an initial ED dose in patients who are later confirmed to have the diagnosis of acute MI. ASA may also

The vast majority of patients admitted for unstable angina should be administered heparin. Exceptions are those on their way to the cardiac catheterization laboratory and patients at low short-term risk of events, such as those without symptoms in the preceding 24 hours despite the diagnosis of new onset angina or change in anginal threshold. Also, there are contraindications to heparin administration, such as recent cerebral hemorrhage or gastrointestinal bleeding. Since heparin can be rapidly reversed with protamine, the risk of minor bleeding needs to be weighed against the potential benefit in a patient at high risk of a cardiac event.

prevent reactivation of acute IHD when heparin therapy is discontinued later in the hospital course. Finally, ASA has demonstrated efficacy in long-term secondary prevention. Heparin, on the other hand, is the most efficacious agent available to reduce early in-hospital ischemic events. Thus, the combination of the two agents for initial therapy in unstable angina is strongly recommended.

Treatment and Assessment of Relief of Symptomatic Ischemia
Treatment of Symptomatic Ischemia.

Recommendation: Anti-ischemia medication should be begun and titrated to dosages that are adequate to relieve symptomatic ischemia without excessive bradycardia or hypotension. Patients should be encouraged to participate in monitoring the success of medication in relieving their pain. Use of a 10-point numerical pain rating scale, visual analog scale, or adjective rating scale is suggested to help them describe the intensity of pain (strength of evidence = C).

Relief of symptoms of unstable angina is attempted in the ED with beta blockers and nitrates. If oral and sublingual administration of these agents does not relieve ischemia, IV use is indicated. Morphine sulfate is used when these measures are ineffective and can also be helpful during the initial stages of therapy while these other agents are being titrated up to target doses. After initial symptom control is achieved, any recurrent ischemic symptoms should prompt performance of an urgent ECG with the goal of obtaining a recording during symptoms. Calcium channel blockers are reserved for patients requiring an additional agent beyond nitrates and beta blockers and for patients with variant angina. The detailed rationale and mode of use for each of these agents are presented in Chapter 4.

Patients who are counseled on the goal of relief of ischemic symptoms can assist greatly in monitoring effectiveness of therapy by accurately reporting changes in pain intensity. Patients with well-developed coping skills may underreport their

Observation of the patient during pain can be extremely useful, especially if done unobtrusively. In addition to direct information regarding the patient's degree of distress, observation provides a basis for judging whether or not the patient is using the 10-point scale appropriately. It is not rare to encounter patients who will report 8 out of 10 chest pain while reading the newspaper. Definite severe distress despite the absence of ECG changes may signal the need for an urgent search for a potentially catastrophic noncardiac etiology for the patient's symptoms, especially aortic dissection and pulmonary embolism.

Although the 10-point pain severity scale is often useful in the initial evaluation of patients, its use should be avoided thereafter for several reasons. Some patients use the scale to manipulate the medical staff to obtain morphine injections and other medications. Some patients misuse the scale after they observe that reporting higher scores causes increased staff attention to them. Also, after the initial diagnosis and treatment are decided, any recurrent discomfort of ischemic etiology is a cause for concern.

pain. In addition, some patients believe that because they are ill, they should expect to feel some pain. These patients often receive less medication than they need to control their anginal symptoms. Use of an objective scale aids in assessment of efficiency of treatment to relieve pain and ischemia. The 10-point individual patient-based intensity score grades pain in severity ranging from 1 being barely perceptible to 10 being the most severe pain ever experienced (Scott and Huskisson, 1976; Sriwatanakul, Kelvie, Lasagna et al., 1983).

Assessment of the Relief of Ischemia.   A vast majority of patients who present with signs of ischemia at rest stabilize rapidly and have decreasing or absent chest pain after 30 minutes of aggressive medical management. These patients should be admitted to an ICU or intermediate care unit. Failure to respond to initial therapy should prompt reconsideration of other possible catastrophic causes of chest pain including ongoing acute MI, aortic dissection, pulmonary embolism, pneumothorax, esophageal rupture, or rupture or ischemia of intra-abdominal organs. Patients considered to have unstable angina after further evaluation who fail to respond within 30 minutes to initial treatment are at increased risk for MI or cardiac death (Gibson, Young, Boden et al., 1987; Larsson, Jonasson, Ringqvist et al., 1992; Silva, Galli, and Campolo, 1993). These patients are best served by care in the ICU of an institution with capabilities to perform intra-aortic balloon pump (IABP) placement, cardiac catheterization, PTCA, and CABG. Transfer may be considered to another institution when ED care has begun in an institution without access to these invasive technologies.

For practical purposes, the physician need only resolve the question of whether immediate cardiac catheterization is indicated; decisions regarding the other interventions mentioned here would be appropriate only after angiography. The only exception is the rare hemodynamically unstable patient in whom an IABP is placed before attempting coronary angiography. However, this is usually best accomplished in the catheterization laboratory, if available.

The benefits of transfer to a facility providing these options of care must be weighed against the risks. In some cases, such as extremely elderly patients or elderly patients with advanced comorbidity, transfer may be inappropriate and/or not in accordance with the wishes of the patient and his or her family. However, in most situations, prompt transfer of severely ill patients with unstable angina to an institution offering definitive care is the most judicious choice. Where long distances are involved, helicopter transport staffed by cardiovascular specialists may benefit deteriorating patients with unstable angina, but ambulance transport is usually adequate in the absence of signs of hemodynamic instability. In remote regions of the country where transfer is not feasible, care should continue in the most satisfactory environment available. Aggressive pharmacologic treatment should continue during the time interval between the decision for transfer, and the time transfer could occur with the option to abort the transfer if the patient improves sufficiently.

Patient Counseling

Recommendation: As permitted by the level of urgency, the health care team should inform the patient and the patient's family or advocate of the probable diagnosis, most reasonable treatment strategies, and most likely outcomes at appropriate intervals during initial evaluation and treatment. At the conclusion of this phase, questions and plans for the next phase of care should be addressed (strength of evidence = C).

The symptoms of unstable angina often develop abruptly, evoking anxiety and fear in patients. Moreover, the prevalence of cardiac death in our society leads many patients to overestimate the potential threat of their cardiac symptoms, and this fear is reinforced by the obvious concern of health care providers. Many patients will be treated by health care providers they do not know, and others lack knowledge of the health care system and its procedures. Good communication between the patient and health care providers is often hindered by these factors and further reduced by the immediate need of the health care team to diagnose and stabilize the patient. Health care providers must overcome communication barriers and provide the patients timely reassurance and information relating to appropriate management of their condition.

Management of patients with unstable angina often requires a decision on the use of alternative tests and procedures with major risks and benefits to patients, and the clinical situation often imposes urgency on reaching these decisions. Obtaining appropriate informed consent is necessary medical practice and is not reiterated at every decision point in this guideline. Patients may be assisted in the difficult task of assimilating and responding appropriately to this information during periods of stress by reiteration of information. The patient may wish to designate a family member or other friend to serve as an advocate for the patient to ensure that the patient understands the information presented by the health care team and to assist in articulating the preferences of the patient. The role of the advocate should not be considered adversarial but should facilitate better communication between care providers and the patient. Communication efforts from health care providers promote a sense of teamwork with the patient and will be rewarded by less anxiety and increased compliance for the patient.

Conclusion of Initial Evaluation and Treatment Phase

At the conclusion of the initial evaluation and treatment phase, the patient presenting with symptoms suggestive of unstable angina should be assigned to one of four diagnostic categories:

1. Alternate diagnosis, not IHD.
2. Stable angina.
3. Reperfusion-eligible acute MI.
4. Unstable angina.

In assigning patients to these groups, the general approach should be to assume that the patient's symptoms are due to CAD until proven otherwise.

Patients with a diagnosis other than unstable angina and patients with known CAD who are felt to have symptoms attributable to another cause are managed as indicated by their presumptive diagnoses. Patients with suspected unstable angina, but with symptoms that are not sufficiently severe to meet definitional criteria for unstable angina, are categorized and managed as stable angina. Patients with prolonged (i.e., >20 minutes) chest discomfort and ECG evidence of epicardial injury (ST-segment elevation or ST-segment depression described in Chapters 3, 4, and 5 of this guideline.

Recommendation: High-risk unstable angina patients should be admitted initially to an ICU bed whenever possible (strength of evidence = B). Intermediate-risk unstable angina patients should be admitted to an ICU or monitored cardiac bed (strength of evidence = C). Low-risk unstable angina

As discussed above, many unstable angina patients are admitted to sub-acute care beds-monitored, 1:4 nurse to patient ratio, and ACLS capability. Few unstable angina patients are admitted to standard floor beds unless they are low-risk patients admitted because of geographic isolation or treatment of comorbidities. Thus, the issue becomes whom to admit to the ICU/CCU.

patients may be managed as outpatients with planned early followup evaluations (strength of evidence = C).

Selection of the appropriate environment for further care of patients diagnosed as having unstable angina is determined primarily by assessment of the short-term risk of untoward events. This benefit must be balanced against the extra monetary cost and possibility of complications from needlessly intensive care (Wears, Li, Hernandez et al., 1989). High-risk patients should be admitted to an ICU environment and ideally should be kept there until they have been stabilized and are symptom-free for at least 24 hours or additional prognostic information is obtained (e.g., resting measure of LV function, acute coronary angiography) that indicates they are not as high risk as initially believed. Patients judged intermediate risk may occasionally be managed by careful, intense outpatient care, but more commonly will be admitted to an ICU, intermediate care unit, or monitored hospital bed (Fineberg, Scadden, and Goldman, 1984). At this transition point, intermediate- and high-risk patients should have a basic understanding of what will happen in the next 3 to 6 hours, including knowledge of the identity of the physicians and nurses with primary care responsibility. Low-risk patients who retain the working, but not definite, diagnosis of unstable angina after initial evaluation should undergo additional evaluation as soon as can be arranged but generally no later than 72 hours after initial presentation.

Medical Record

Information to be entered in the medical record summarizing initial evaluation and management for each patient includes:

- Age and sex.
- Duration and nature of symptoms prior to presentation.
- Previous history of CAD: if yes, prior noninvasive test result, prior cardiac catheterization result, prior myocardial revascularization procedure (bypass or angioplasty).
- Medication and drug use.
- Risk factors (diabetes, smoking, hypercholesterolemia, hypertension).
- Systemic causes for precipitating or exacerbating ischemia.

Table 15.   Criteria for ICU/CCU admission

Severe hypoxia/intubation
Severe hypotension/shock/IABP
Suspected acute MI
Uncontrolled arrhythmias
Tamponade
Serious comorbidity (sepsis, renal failure)
Very high risk for an event

- ECG interpretation.
- Initial and final assignment of likelihood of CAD (high, intermediate, low) and basis.
- Initial and final risk assignment (high, intermediate, low) and basis.
- Summary of other pertinent positive and negative findings.
- Major or minor complications of diagnosis or treatment.
- Patient counseling, including assessment of patient response.
- Disposition for further care.
- Deaths classified as noncardiac or cardiac.
- Cardiac deaths classified as precipitated by arrhythmia, progressive ischemia, or progressive cardiac failure.

Duration of Initial Evaluation and Treatment Phase

The initial assessment of whether a patient has unstable angina and which triage option is most suitable generally should be made within the first hour after the patient's arrival at a medical facility. Lack of appropriate hospital beds or transport facilities to move the patient to another medical facility may prevent expedient implementation of the triage decision. In such cases, stabilization and management of ischemic symptoms should continue as if the patient were admitted to the hospital. Patients judged to be low risk at initial evaluation may have completion of their definitive evaluation deferred for up to 72 hours as long as the severity and frequency of symptoms do not worsen.

3

Guideline: Outpatient Care

Commentary by Michael H. Crawford, M.D.

Introduction

Patients with unstable angina who are judged in the initial evaluation and treatment phase to be at low risk for adverse outcomes can, in many cases, be safely evaluated further as outpatients. Typically, these are patients who have experienced new onset or worsening symptoms that may be due to ischemia, but they have not had severe, prolonged, or rest episodes in the preceding 2 weeks. Their followup evaluation should have been scheduled as soon as possible, generally 72 hours after the initial presentation. In addition, patients with symptoms suggestive of unstable angina whose presentations are not considered sufficiently urgent to require ED evaluation may be seen first in an outpatient facility. This chapter addresses care of patients presenting for initial evaluation as well as those patients who had initial evaluation in an ED (usually within the past 72 hours) and now present for more definitive evaluation of possible unstable angina (see Figure 6).

Objectives of Care

In patients without known CAD, the three goals of outpatient care are to assess further the cause of the patient's symptoms, evaluate the risk of future adverse cardiac events, and provide adequate symptom relief. In patients with known CAD, the primary concern is whether to intensify medical therapy or consider PTCA or CABG.

Approach to Care Objectives

Diagnostic Assessment

All patients should have a history, physical examination, and ECG. Initial evaluation for patients without prior ED evaluation should proceed as described for low-risk patients in Chapter 2. For patients returning for followup examination of a recent ED visit, the circumstances surrounding the initial presentation and any interval symptoms since the initial examination represent the important features of the history. Evidence of a worsening symptom pattern may necessitate hospital admission for control and further diagnostic workup. This repeat evaluation should also include a further search for factors that might precipitate or exacerbate unstable angina, such as fever, tachyarrhythmias, hyperthyroidism, severe anemia, cocaine use, noncompliance with medical therapy, environmental temperature extremes, severe psychosocial stress, and changes in the level of physical exertion or lifestyle.

Patients who develop pain during the clinic visit should have a careful cardiac examination during the episode (looking for a new S_4 or S_3, new or worsening MR murmur, rales) and an immediate ECG (looking for transient changes in the ST-segment or T-wave). A therapeutic trial with sublingual NTG can be attempted after these steps if the discomfort is still present. Repeat examination and an ECG should be performed once symptoms are completely resolved.

Risk Stratification and Further Management

Recommendation: Exercise or pharmacologic stress testing generally should be part of the detailed outpatient workup. However, patients found to have high-risk features (see Table 9), such as evidence of significant LV dysfunction, or an interval acceleration or worsening of symptoms while on appropriate levels of medical therapy, should be considered for direct referral to cardiac catheterization. In addition, patients who have symptoms felt very unlikely to be due to CAD or who are felt to be at very low risk for cardiac events can be managed conservatively, with stress testing reserved for recurrent or worsening symptoms (strength of evidence = C).

After detailed clinical assessment, the clinician will have formed an estimate of the likelihood of CAD (see Table 8) and will have made a clinical judgment of the risk of short-term adverse events (see Table 9). Patients found to have high-risk features, especially those with evidence of LV dysfunction or CHF, should be considered for prompt ICU admission for intensive medical care (see Chapter 4). Patients who have a low likelihood of CAD and are at low risk may benefit by further evaluation that may include a trial of nitrates and beta blockers. Use of noninvasive testing in this population should be delayed until the clinical presentation is more clear to avoid the anxiety and cost associated with the false-positive test common in this low-risk population. In general, all intermediate-risk patients and low-risk patients with an intermediate or high likelihood of CAD benefit from noninvasive testing. A more complete discussion of noninvasive testing in this patient group is included in Chapter 6.

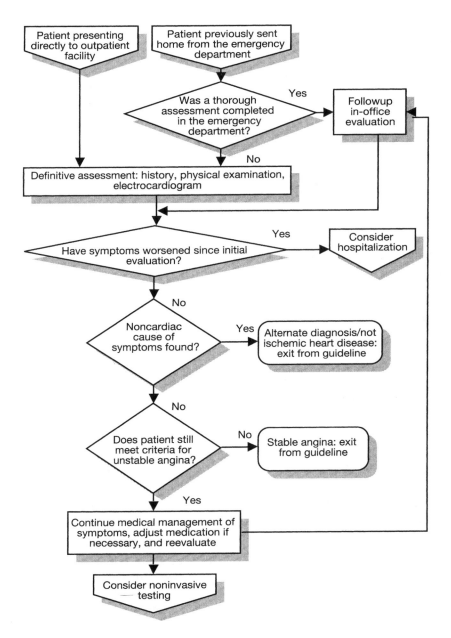

Figure 6. Patient flow: Outpatient care.

Outpatient care is directed at those patients who are not admitted. These are mainly low-risk patients with an intermediate likelihood of disease or low-risk patients with a low likelihood of disease, since most patients with intermediate risk and intermediate likelihood of coronary disease would be admitted. The major rule of outpatient care promulgated by the guideline is that an evaluation of the patient must be completed within 72 hours. The principal form of evaluation recommended is a stress test. The guideline states that most outpatients should be evaluated by stress testing, but certainly all patients at intermediate risk with a low likelihood of coronary disease, and patients at low risk with an intermediate or high likelihood of coronary disease should be tested. Interestingly, they recommend that patients with a low likelihood of coronary disease and a low estimated risk should not be evaluated by any test. The evidence in support of this recommendation was graded at level C. It would be unwise to follow this recommendation, since it would unnecessarily expose one to litigation. The cost of an exercise stress test, especially in a patient with a normal ECG in whom a nonimaging test can be done, is low enough that the extra assuredness provided is well worth it for the patient's and the physician's peace of mind.

The guideline recommends outpatient cardiac catheterization only for those patients with demonstrated LV dysfunction, an increase in symptoms, an increase in medicines from the ED, or patients at high risk of an event or who are not reassured by a negative stress test. The last recommendation for cardiac catheterization is rather vague and could be subject to manipulation by the physician. However, patients certainly do exist who need to know their anatomy and are quite insistent.

Outpatient Treatment of Symptoms

Recommendation: Patients should be instructed in the proper use of sublingual NTG tablets (strength of evidence = C).

Recommendation: Medical therapy for presumed CAD usually begins with sublingual NTG, followed by oral beta blockers. Long-acting topical or oral nitrates may be added, but care should be taken to use regimens that reduce the likelihood of tolerance. In general, for low-risk outpatients, therapy with ASA and one antianginal medication is sufficient initial treatment unless patients have additional indications for multiagent therapy (e.g., hypertension, supraventricular arrhythmia) (strength of evidence = C). Long-acting forms of antianginal drugs are preferable to enhance patient compliance (strength of evidence = C).

This regimen is probably less expensive than starting a patient on a calcium blocker, although one calcium blocker may do the job of a beta blocker-nitrate combination with regard to controlling symptoms. Although not discussed in this section of the guideline, dihydropyridine calcium blockers are contraindicated in unstable angina, because of unfavorable outcome experience in large clinical trials. It is believed that the so-called rate lowering calcium blockers, such as diltiazem and verapamil, are safer, especially if the patient has no evidence of LV dysfunction or heart block. These more costly drugs are certainly discouraged in the guideline despite the fact that beta blockers and long-acting nitrates are frequently associated with significant side effects. Interestingly, a recent evaluation of the experience at a large Chicago institution showed that the lack of beta-blocker or calcium-blocker use prior to admission predicted the occurrence of major cardiac complications in the hospital (Calvin et al., 1995). Other factors also of independent predictive value on multivariate analysis were need for IV NTG, prior MI < 14 days ago, baseline ST-segment depression, diabetes, and age.

Recommendation: Patients with established CAD who are already on medical therapy should have their medical regimen reviewed and dosages increased as appropriate and as tolerated (strength of evidence = C).

Recommendation: Patients with established CAD or who are judged to be intermediate or high likelihood for CAD should be maintained on ASA at 160 to 324 mg per day unless contraindications are present (strength of evidence = A, evidence cited in Chapter 2). Patients unable to take ASA because of a history of true hypersensitivity or recent significant GI bleeding may be started on ticlopidine 250 mg twice per day as a substitute (strength of evidence = B, evidence cited in Chapter 4).

The symptomatic therapy of patients with low-risk unstable angina not requiring hospitalization involves the use of sublingual NTG for treatment of individual anginal episodes and prophylactic therapy with an agent from one of the three major classes of antianginal drugs (nitrates, beta blockers, calcium antagonists). In general, it is reasonable to start therapy with one major antianginal, preferably in a long-acting preparation, and proceed to a second agent only if there are recurrent symptoms on optimal doses of the first agent. In addition, ASA should be a standard part of each regimen. The details of these therapies and the evidence for their use are described in Chapter 4.

Recommendation: Patients who continue to report symptoms they consider to reflect cardiac disease and are not reassured that they do not have CAD by

Another issue in the outpatient management of patients with unstable angina is what to do with the patient with known CAD. Should one merely increase their medications or proceed to cardiac catheterization followed by revascularization? The guideline suggest increasing medications, unless the patient meets the criteria for an invasive approach. It makes sense to increase the dosage of the patient's antianginal drugs to maximally tolerated levels. Although it is tempting to escalate unstable angina patients to maximum all-class multidrug therapy, evidence suggests that this may not be necessary. The use of multiple drugs increases the cost of therapy and usually the incidence of side effects. A recent study has shown that the effectiveness of combination drug therapy in patients with angina pectoris is most often due to recruitment of patients not responding to maximum monotherapy, rather than any synergistic or additive effect. (Savonitto et al., 1996) Thus, if the patient is still symptomatic on maximum doses of one class of drug (monotherapy), in general a new drug class should be substituted for rather than added to the first. Only if symptoms are partially controlled by one drug should a second be added.

appropriate noninvasive tests, counseling, and rehabilitation may be candidates for cardiac catheterization to confirm the absence of CAD (strength of evidence = C).

Some patients who present with symptoms suggestive of unstable angina and are initially categorized as having low likelihood of CAD will continue to report symptoms suggestive of angina despite an antianginal regimen that appears appropriate. The medical provider should first review all diagnoses and management decisions and, if appropriate, obtain or repeat other noninvasive exercise or pharmacologic stress tests. Fear of heart disease or other psychological problems commonly underlie complaints of cardiovascular symptoms which are out of proportion to objective evidence of ischemia. Some patients benefit from more complete and frequent counseling and reassurance. This group of patients will often respond to cardiac rehabilitation in a structured environment with supervised exercise. A trial of simple measures is reasonable in this group of patients, but failure to respond may necessitate the decision to perform a cardiac catheterization with the intention of confirming the absence of coronary artery disease. If this is to be undertaken, patients must be informed of the reason for the procedure when they provide informed consent.

Some patients find sufficient reassurance with angiographic documentation of normal coronary arteries that their symptoms gradually dissipate. Patients who continue to have symptoms they consider to be angina despite normal coronary angiograms may have small-vessel or vasospastic CAD requiring further evaluation that is not covered by this guideline. Other patients with continued symptoms but no objective evidence of ischemia or CAD may benefit from evaluation and counseling by medical practitioners other than cardiovascular specialists.

Patient Counseling

Patients and their families and advocates should understand the most likely diagnosis at the conclusion of the outpatient evaluation. Discussion should deal directly with clinical and test results that predict risk and possible outcomes. Further evaluation and treatment options should be discussed. Patients should receive from the doctor, nurse, or pharmacist a clear explanation of the rationale for use of medicines and suggested dosages, as well as possible side effects. On return visits, patients should be asked about their reaction and compliance as well as perceived effectiveness of the treatment plan outlined on the prior visit. All patients should be counseled on risk-factor modification.

Medical Record

Information that should be updated or added to the medical record at the conclusion of outpatient management includes:

- Age and sex.
- Duration and nature of symptoms prior to presentation.
- Previous history of CAD: if yes, prior noninvasive test result, cardiac catheterization result, and/or myocardial revascularization procedure (bypass or angioplasty).
- Medication and drug use.
- Risk factors (diabetes, smoking, hypercholesterolemia, hypertension).
- Systemic causes for precipitating or exacerbating ischemia.
- ECG interpretation.
- Initial and final assignment of likelihood of CAD (high, intermediate, low) and basis.
- Initial and final risk assignment (high, intermediate, low) and basis.
- Summary of other pertinent positive and negative findings.
- Patient counseling, including assessment of patient response.
- Disposition for further care.
- Results of ancillary clinical studies.
- Final diagnosis.
- Final disposition.
- Effectiveness of antianginal medication used.

Duration of Outpatient Phase

Typically, the interval between initial presentation and initiation of comprehensive outpatient evaluation should be no more than 72 hours. Generally, one clinic visit should be sufficient to establish a working diagnosis, assess risk, and develop a management plan. Serial outpatient evaluation and noninvasive testing may be required depending on the patient's specific findings and response to treatment. Patients with specific indications may be referred for outpatient or inpatient cardiac catheterization.

4

Guideline: Intensive Medical Management

Commentary by Michael H. Crawford, M.D.

Introduction

During the first hour of evaluation and management, the clinician forms an initial assessment of the patient's problem, institutes initial therapeutic steps, and formulates a triage plan, as described in Chapter 2. High-risk and some intermediate-risk patients with unstable angina, including those with ongoing ischemia refractory to initial medical therapy and those with evidence of hemodynamic instability, should be admitted to an ICU environment with ready access to invasive cardiovascular diagnosis and therapy. This patient group will include some patients with undiagnosed acute MI, but patients with acute MI manifesting ST-segment elevation will have been excluded during initial evaluation. Details of ICU management, early laboratory testing, and risk stratification for these patients are discussed in this chapter (see Figure 7).

Objectives of Care

Two of the major goals of this phase are to relieve pain and ischemia and to plan a definitive treatment strategy for the underlying disease process. A few patients will require prompt triage to emergency or urgent cardiac catheterization and/or placement of an IABP. However, most patients usually stabilize after a brief period of intensive pharmacologic management and, after appropriate counseling, will choose an approach for definitive therapy. Some patients will choose a more invasive strategy that may involve cardiac catheterization, PTCA, or CABG. Other patients will prefer continuation or initiation of an integrated medical regimen. These patients require careful monitoring of the response to initial therapy with surveillance for ischemia or other complications of unstable angina that may require a change in approach to treatment.

Approach to Care Objectives

Pharmacologic Management

Nitrates.

Recommendation: Patients whose symptoms are not fully relieved with three sublingual NTG tablets and initiation of beta-blocker therapy (when possible), as well as all nonhypotensive high-risk unstable angina patients, may benefit from IV NTG, and such therapy is recommended in the absence of contraindications. IV NTG should be started at a dose of 5 to 10 μg/min by continuous infusion and titrated up by 10 μg/min every 5 to 10 minutes until relief of symptoms or limiting side effects (headache or hypotension with SBP <90 mmHg or more than 30 percent below starting mean arterial pressure levels if significant hypertension is present) (strength of evidence = B). Topical, oral, or buccal nitrates are acceptable alternatives for patients without ongoing or refractory symptoms (strength of evidence = B).

Recommendation: Patients on IV NTG should be switched to oral or topical nitrate therapy once they have been symptom-free for 24 hours (strength of evidence = C). Tolerance to nitrates is dose- and duration-dependent and typically becomes significant only after 24 hours of continuous therapy. Responsiveness to nitrates can be restored by increasing the dose or switching the patient to a nonparenteral form of therapy and using a nitrate-free interval. As long as the patient's symptoms are not adequately controlled, the former option should be selected. Topical, oral, or buccal nitrates should be given with a 6- to 8-hour nitrate-free interval (strength of evidence = C).

NTG has both peripheral and coronary vascular effects. It increases venous pooling, thereby decreasing myocardial preload and LV-end diastolic volume. The more modest effects on the arterial circulation are not believed to be a major contributor to the therapeutic effect of NTG. NTG vasodilates normal and atherosclerotic coronary arteries and promotes coronary collateral flow. In severe coronary obstruction, physiologic responses to decreased myocardial blood flow promote maximal vasodilatation in the absence of drug therapy. Thus, the primary benefit of NTG in unstable angina is believed to be due to decreased preload with consequent reduction in myocardial oxygen demand. Recently, an inhibition of platelet aggregation effect has been reported, but it is uncertain if this contributes to clinical benefits.

Most studies of IV NTG in unstable angina have been small and uncontrolled (Depace, Herling, Kotler et al., 1982; Distante, Maseri, Severi et al., 1979; Kaplan, Davison, Parker et al., 1983; Roubin, Harris, Eckhardt et al., 1982). There are no randomized placebo controlled trials in unstable angina that address either the efficacy of the drug in symptom relief or reduction of cardiac events. One small randomized trial compared IV NTG with buccal NTG and found no significant difference (Dellborg, Gustafsson, and Swedberg, 1991). Pooled analysis of studies of

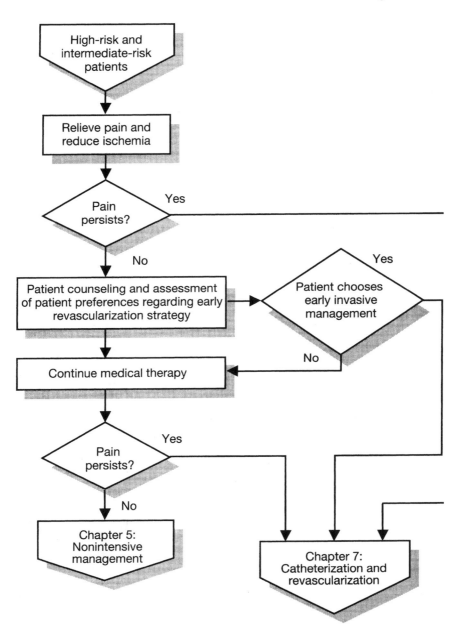

Figure 7. Patient flow: Intensive medical management.

NTG in patients with acute MI from the prethrombolytic era suggest a 35 percent reduction in mortality (Yusuf, Collins, MacMahon et al., 1988). However, the ISIS-4 (*Lancet* 1995; 345: 669–85) and GISSI-3 trials (Lancet 1994; 343; 1115–22) in acute MI patients receiving thrombolytic therapy failed to confirm this benefit. Abrupt ce$acssation of IV NTG has been associated with exacerbation of ischemic changes on ECG (Figueras, Lidon, and Cortadellas, 1991).

Thus, the rationale for the use of this agent in unstable angina is extrapolated from pathophysiologic principles, uncontrolled studies of efficacy, beneficial effects on mortality in acute MI, and clinical experience. There are no data that define the proper timing of initiation of therapy or its useful duration. Considerable evidence has now accumulated that continuous administration of nitrates can lead to attenuation or even elimination of therapeutic effect in as few as 24 hours (May, Popma, and Black, 1987; Reichek, Priest, Zimrin et al., 1984; Thadani, Hamilton, Olsen et al., 1986). Consequently, nitrates should be given with a nitrate-free period when topical, buccal, or oral nitrates are administered. In addition, in stabilized patients, IV NTG should generally be converted within 72 hours to a nonparenteral alternative to avoid attenuation of effects and potential reactivation of symptoms. Patients who require continued IV NTG beyond 24 hours may require periodic increases in infusion rate to maintain efficacy.

Morphine Sulfate.

Recommendation: Morphine sulfate at a dose of 2 to 5 mg IV is recommended for any patient whose symptoms are not relieved after three serial sublingual NTG tablets or whose symptoms recur with adequate anti-ischemic therapy unless contraindicated by hypotension or intolerance. Morphine may be repeated every 5 to 30 minutes as needed to relieve symptoms and maintain patient comfort (strength of evidence = C).

Morphine sulfate has potent analgesic and anxiolytic effects, as well as hemodynamic effects, that are potentially beneficial in unstable angina. Meperidine hydrochloride can be substituted for morphine in patients who are allergic to morphine. No randomized trials have defined the unique contribution of morphine to the initial therapeutic regimen or its optimal administration schedule. However, morphine has many beneficial properties in unstable angina, including relief of pain and anxiety and decreases in cardiac work and oxygen consumption. In particular, morphine causes significant venodilation. In addition, it may produce modest reductions in heart rate (through increased vagal tone) and SBP. The major adverse reaction to morphine in unstable angina is an exaggeration of its therapeutic effect causing significant hypotension, especially in the presence of concomitant vasodilator therapy. This problem usually responds to IV saline boluses; rarely, pressors or naloxone may be required to restore an adequate blood pressure. The other frequent adverse reactions are nausea and vomiting, which occur in 20 percent or more of patients. Respiratory depression is the most serious complica-

IV NTG is considered the mainstay of therapy for ongoing ischemic chest pain. In fact, morphine is rarely used, unless maximum doses of IV NTG are not controlling the pain. Since there is no evidence that nitrates have any special therapeutic or prophylactic value in unstable angina, they should only be given to patients with symptoms. Some physicians give nitrates to all patients admitted with ischemic heart disease, regardless of symptoms. However, since nitrates can cause hypotension, aggravation of myocardial ischemia, and other adverse events, this practice should be discouraged. IV nitrates are usually given until the short-term therapeutic goals for the patient are determined. If the patient is going on medical therapy, then the IV nitrates are stopped and oral agents substituted. If the patient is going on to a revascularization procedure, usually the nitrates are continued until that procedure is accomplished. There are some exceptions to not using NTG in asymptomatic CAD patients. Nitrates can be useful for lowering hypertensive blood pressure values and can help reduce preload in patients with congestive heart failure. However, there are other more specific and potent agents for these purposes.

tion of morphine; severe respiratory hypoventilation requiring intubation occurs in only about 1 percent of acute IHD patients treated with this agent.

Beta Blockers.

Recommendation: IV (for high-risk patients) or oral (for intermediate- and low-risk patients) beta blockers should be started in the absence of contraindications (strength of evidence = B).

Recommendation: Choice of the specific agent is not as important as ensuring that appropriate candidates receive this therapy. If there are concerns about patient intolerance due to existing pulmonary disease, especially asthma, LV dysfunction, or risk of hypotension or severe bradycardia, initial selection should favor a short-acting agent, such as propranolol or metoprolol or the ultra short-acting agent esmolol. Mild wheezing or a history of COPD should prompt a trial of a short-acting agent at a reduced dose (e.g., 2.5 mg IV metoprolol, 12.5 mg oral metoprolol, or 25 μg/kg/min esmolol as initial doses) rather than complete avoidance of beta-blocker therapy (strength of evidence = C).

Recommendation: IV metoprolol is given in 5 mg increments by slow (over 1 to 2 minutes) IV administration repeated every 5 minutes for a total initial dose of 15 mg followed in 1 to 2 hours by 25 to 50 mg by mouth every 6 hours.

If a very conservative regimen is desired with metoprolol, initial doses can be reduced to 1 to 2 mg. IV propranolol is given as an initial dose of 0.5 to 1.0 mg, followed in 1 to 2 hours by 40 to 80 mg by mouth every 6 to 8 hours. IV esmolol is given as a starting maintenance dose of 0.1 mg/kg/min with titration in increments of 0.05 mg/kg/min every 10 to 15 minutes as tolerated by blood pressure until the desired therapeutic response has been obtained, limiting symptoms develop, or a dose of 0.20 mg/kg/min is reached. An optional loading dose of 0.5 mg/kg may be given by slow IV administration (2 to 5 minutes) for more rapid onset of action. In patients suitable for a longer acting agent, IV atenolol can be initiated with a 5 mg IV dose followed 5 minutes later by a second 5 mg IV dose and then 50 to 100 mg orally per day initiated 1 to 2 hours after the IV dose. Monitoring during IV beta-blocker therapy should include frequent checks of heart rate and blood pressure and continuous ECG monitoring, as well as auscultation for rales or bronchospasm. After the initial IV load, patients without limiting side effects may be converted to an oral regimen. The target heart rate for beta blockade is 50 to 60 beats per minute. Selection of the oral agent should be based on the clinician's familiarity with the agent as well as the risk of adverse effects (strength of evidence = C).

Beta-blocking agents are competitive antagonists to catecholamines which exert their effects at cell membrane beta receptors. Beta[1] receptors are located primarily in the myocardium; inhibition of catecholamine action at these sites reduces cardiac contractility, sinus node rate, and AV node conduction velocity. Beta[2] receptors are located primarily in vascular and bronchial smooth muscle; inhibition of catecholamine action at these sites produces arterial vasoconstriction and bronchoconstriction. In unstable angina, the primary benefits of beta-blocker therapy are due to its effects on beta[1] receptors that decrease cardiac work and myocardial oxygen demand.

Initial studies of beta-blocker benefits in acute IHD were small and uncontrolled. Three double-blind randomized trials have compared beta blockers to placebo in unstable angina (Gottlieb, Weisfeldt, Ouyang et al., 1986; Lubsen and Tijssen, 1987; Telford and Wilson, 1981). Meta-analysis of the available trials indicates a 13 percent reduction in risk of progression to acute MI (Yusuf, Wittes, and Friedman, 1988). No clear effect on mortality in unstable angina has been shown to date. However, randomized trials in acute MI, recent MI, and stable angina with silent ischemia have all shown a mortality benefit for beta blockers. Thus, the overall rationale for the use of beta blockers is compelling and sufficient to make them a routine part of care for patients with unstable angina in the absence of contraindications.

Choice of beta blocker for an individual patient is based primarily on pharmacokinetic and side-effect criteria. There is no evidence that any member of this class of agents is more effective in producing beneficial effects in unstable angina

All studies in unstable angina have shown that beta blockers significantly reduce the incidence of subsequent MI, and thus, their use in unstable angina is strongly encouraged. The major problem with these agents is the contraindications to their use and the frequent occurrence of adverse effects. Thus, given that they do not change overall mortality, many physicians are more circumspect in their use. IV beta blockade is rarely used in unstable angina, unless the patient has marked tachycardia or hypertension, or if acute MI is suspected. Also, if beta blockers are believed to be beneficial for the patient, but the physician is afraid to use them because of potential adverse effects, IV esmolol is a good way to test the patient's tolerance to beta blockers.

than any other. The specific benefits and disadvantages of using an agent with intrinsic sympathomimetic activity remain unsettled. On the basis of side-effect profiles, initial choice of agents favors metoprolol or atenolol, and esmolol can be used if a continuous infusion is required (e.g., patient is unable to take oral medication).

Patients with marked 1° atrioventricular (AV) block (i.e., ECG PR segment [PR] >0.24 seconds), any form of 2° or 3° AV block, a history of asthma, or severe LV dysfunction with CHF or cardiogenic shock should not receive beta blockers. Patients with significant sinus bradycardia (heart rate <60 beats/min) or hypotension (SBP <90 mmHg) generally should not receive beta blockers until these conditions have resolved. Patients with significant COPD that may have a component of reactive airway disease should be given beta blockers cautiously; initially, low doses of a beta[1] selective agent should be used.

In summary, evidence for the beneficial effects of beta blockers in unstable angina is based on limited randomized trial data, along with pathophysiologic considerations and extrapolation from experience with stable angina and acute MI. The recommendation for IV beta blockers in high-risk patients is based on the demonstrated benefit in acute MI patients, as well as the hemodynamic objectives of therapy to reduce cardiac work and myocardial oxygen demand. The duration of benefit with long-term oral therapy is uncertain but appears in the acute MI literature to extend out for at least 5 years.

Calcium Channel Blockers.

Recommendation: Calcium channel blockers may be used to control ongoing or recurring ischemic symptoms in patients already on adequate doses of nitrates and beta blockers or in patients unable to tolerate adequate doses of one or both of these agents or in patients with variant angina (strength of evidence = B). Calcium channel blockers should be avoided in patients with pulmonary edema or evidence of LV dysfunction (strength of evidence = B).

Choice of individual calcium channel blocker is based primarily on the hemodynamic state of the patient, risk of adverse effects on contractility and AV conduction, and the clinician's familiarity with available agents (strength of evidence = C). Nifedipine should not be used in the absence of concurrent beta blockade (strength of evidence = A).

Calcium channel blockers reduce the myocardial cell transmembrane inward flux of calcium which in turn affects myocardial and vascular smooth muscle contraction, as well as AV conduction. The agents in this class vary in the degree to which they produce clinically important vasodilation, decreased myocardial contractility, and increased AV block. Nifedipine and amlodipine have the largest peripheral arterial vasodilatory effect, verapamil is intermediate, and diltiazem has the least effect. All four agents appear to have coronary vasodilatory properties that are equivalent. Although the different members of this class of agents are structurally diverse and may have somewhat different mechanisms of action, no reliable data demonstrate superiority of one agent over another in unstable angina. Beneficial effects in unstable angina are believed due to variable combinations of decreased myocardial oxygen demand relating to decreased afterload, contractility, and heart rate. Major side effects relate to exaggeration of these three therapeutic effects: hypotension, worsening CHF, AV block. These agents may also have a beneficial effect on LV diastolic relaxation and compliance.

There are several small randomized trials involving use of a calcium channel blocker in unstable angina. Generally, they show efficacy in relieving symptoms that appears equivalent to beta blockers (Theroux, Taeymans, Morissette et al., 1985). The largest randomized trial, the Holland Interuniversity Trial, tested nifedipine and metoprolol in a 2 × 2 factorial design (Lubsen and Tijssen, 1987). Nifedipine alone increased the risk of MI or recurrent angina relative to placebo by 16 percent, metoprolol decreased it by 24 percent, and the combination of metoprolol and nifedipine was associated with a 20 percent reduction in these events. None of these effects, however, was statistically significant. A meta-analysis of the effects of calcium channel blockers on death or nonfatal MI in unstable angina showed no effect (Held, Yusuf, and Furberg, 1989; Yusuf, Wittes, and Friedman, 1988).

In summary, evidence for the beneficial effects of calcium channel blockers in unstable angina is predominantly limited to control of symptoms (Gerstenblith, Ouyang, Achuff et al., 1982; Muller, Turi, Pearle et al., 1984). The limited randomized trial data available are not consistent with a beneficial effect on mortality or recurrent infarction. In addition, results from randomized trials involving the use of these agents in acute MI patients suggest an overall detrimental effect on mortality, with patients with LV dysfunction being particularly at risk. Thus, this guideline recommends reserving these drugs as second- or third-line therapy following initiation of nitrates and beta blockers. When required for refractory symptom control, these agents can be used during the early in-hospital phase even in pa-

> Calcium blockers are usually not necessary, since most patients can be controlled by IV NTG and beta blockers. Also, many patients with a history of ischemic heart disease or hypertension are already on calcium channel blockers. In these cases, their dose may need to be increased. Perhaps 20 percent of patients not already on calcium blockers will eventually need them to control their symptomatology. However, usually calcium blockers are added during the transition from IV NTG to oral medications. Calcium blockers are often preferred to long-term nitrate therapy, because of a lack of tolerance, fewer side effects, and the ease of once-a-day dosing as compared to isosorbide dinitrate, which must be given 3 times a day. Because of the reports of increased MI using the short-acting dihydropyridines, these drugs are rarely given to patients with unstable angina, even if they are on beta blockers. Rather, diltiazem or verapamil are preferred, unless the patient has LV dysfunction, significant bradycardia, or conduction abnormalities. In patients with contraindications to diltiazem or verapamil who need calcium blocker therapy, it would make sense to use amlodipine, which has not been implicated in any adverse events in unstable angina patients.

tients with LV dysfunction. However, it should be a goal, particularly in the latter group, to replace this therapy with alternatives as promptly as possible. The risks and benefits of amlodipine relative to other agents in this class remain undefined.

Aspirin.

Recommendation: ASA to be taken once per day at a dose of 80 to 324 mg should be continued indefinitely following presentation with unstable angina (strength of evidence = A).

ASA therapy will have been initiated in all patients without contraindications at the time of initial evaluation (see Chapter 2). These patients should be carefully followed for adverse reactions (gastrointestinal upset and bleeding for ASA, thrombocytopenia and bleeding for heparin). The benefit of ASA appears to be sustained when therapy is continued for 1 to 2 years following the initial presentation. Longer term followup data in this particular population are lacking, but given the relatively short-term prognostic impact of unstable angina in coronary disease patients, long-term efficacy can be extrapolated from other studies of ASA therapy in coronary disease. Patients should be informed of the strength of evidence supporting ASA use in unstable angina and CAD. Otherwise, this simple but effective treatment may be discounted by patients because of its low cost and common use for other reasons (e.g., headache, fever).

Ticlopidine and Other Antiplatelet Agents.

Recommendation: Patients unable to take ASA because of a history of hypersensitivity or major GI intolerance may be started on ticlopidine 250 mg twice per day as a substitute (strength of evidence = B).

A small percentage of the unstable angina population is unable to tolerate ASA therapy due to either hypersensitivity (primarily manifesting as life-threatening asthma) or major GI contraindications, principally a recent significant bleed from a peptic ulcer. For these patients, ticlopidine represents a reasonable alternative form of antiplatelet therapy. The mechanism of the antiplatelet effects of ticlopidine remains incompletely defined, is clearly different from ASA, and may include inhibition of mobilization of the fibrinogen receptor in activated platelets.

A multicenter randomized trial of 625 patients in Italy reported a 47 percent reduction in cardiovascular death and a 46 percent reduction in nonfatal MI at 6 months with the use of ticlopidine in unstable angina (Balsano, Rizzon, Violi et al., 1990). This trial did not employ either heparin or ASA, and no comparison of these agents with ticlopidine was performed. For this reason, ticlopidine cannot be recommended as first-line therapy in unstable angina.

Since it takes up to 3 days for the maximal antiplatelet effect of ticlopidine to be achieved, there is no rationale for acute ED administration, as with ASA. Initial treatment with heparin is especially important in those patients with delayed onset of antiplatelet activity. Adverse effects of ticlopidine include GI problems (diarrhea, abdominal pain, nausea, vomiting) and neutropenia (>1,200 neutrophils/mm^3, prevalence approximately 2.4%; severe neutropenia in 0.8%). The latter problem usually resolves within 1 to 3 weeks of discontinuing therapy. Monitoring of ticlopidine therapy includes a complete blood count and differential counts every 2 weeks for the first 3 months of therapy.

A number of other antiplatelet drugs are currently available, and still others are under active investigation. None of the currently available agents, including sulfinpyrazone and dipyridamole, have demonstrated efficacy in unstable angina; for this reason, they cannot be recommended at this time. Current investigational agents that may eventually prove to be more efficacious than ASA include drugs that reversibly block the platelet IIb IIIa receptor.

Recommendation: Heparin infusion should be continued for 2 to 5 days or until revascularization is performed (strength of evidence = C).

Initial heparin dosage is 80 units/kg bolus and IV infusion of 18 units/kg/hour. An aPTT is obtained 6 hours after beginning infusion with the goal of keeping the aPTT between 46 and 70 seconds (Raschke, Reilly, Guidry et al., 1993) or approximately 1.5 to 2.5 times control.

For hospitals with a mean control aPTT value of about 30 seconds, heparin dosage can be adjusted in the following manner:

- aPTT <35   80 units/kg bolus, increase drip 4 units/kg/hour

- aPTT 35 to 45   40 units/kg bolus, increase drip 2 units/kg/hour
- aPTT 46 to 70   no change
- aPTT 71 to 90   reduce drip 2 units/kg/hour
- aPTT >90   hold heparin for 1 hour, reduce drip 3 units/kg/hour

An aPTT should be obtained 6 hours after any dosage change and used to adjust heparin infusion until aPTT is therapeutic (1.5 to 2.5 times control). When two consecutive aPTTs are therapeutic, an aPTT may be ordered and heparin adjusted every 24 hours. In addition, a significant change in the patient's clinical condition (e.g., recurrent definite ischemia, bleeding, hypotension) should prompt an immediate aPTT determination.

Serial hemoglobin/hematocrit and platelet measurements are recommended at least daily for the first 3 days of heparin therapy. In addition, any clinically significant bleeding, recurrent symptoms, or hemodynamic instability should prompt an immediate determination. Serial platelet counts are necessary to monitor for heparin-induced thrombocytopenia. Mild thrombocytopenia may occur in 10 to 20 percent of patients receiving heparin and usually appears in the first 1 to 3 days of therapy, while severe thrombocytopenia (platelet count <100,000) occurs in 1 to 2 percent of patients and typically appears after 3 to 5 days of therapy. Thrombocytopenia appears to be less frequent with bovine heparin than with porcine heparin. A rare complication (probably <0.2% incidence) is heparin-induced thrombocytopenia with thrombosis. This catastrophic complication is believed to be immunologically mediated and occurs equally with bovine and porcine heparin. A high clinical suspicion mandates immediate cessation of all heparin therapy (including that used to flush IV lines) pending further evaluation of this syndrome.

Most of the trials evaluating the use of heparin in unstable angina have continued therapy for ≥5 days. The efficacy of shorter infusion regimens thus remains undefined. Evaluation of data from the Montreal Heart Institute randomized trial of heparin and ASA showed a significantly increased reactivation rate after withdrawal of study drug with heparin alone compared with the other three regimens (Theroux, Waters, Lam et al., 1992). The combination of heparin and ASA appears to mitigate this increase although even with ASA, there is hematologic evidence of increased thrombin activity after cessation of IV heparin. Recent uncontrolled observations suggest a reduction in heparin rebound from switching from IV to subcutaneous heparin for several days before stopping the drug.

Laboratory Testing

Recommendation: Total CK and CK-MB should be measured every 6 to 8 hours for the first 24 hours after admission (strength of evidence = B).

Recommendation: Serial lactate dehydrogenase (LDH) isoenzymes may be useful in detecting myocardial damage in patients presenting between 24 and

Heparin is one of the mainstays of unstable angina treatment and should be given to almost all patients, unless there is a contraindication. Many unstable angina studies from other countries report giving heparin for ≥5 days, but this is not possible in most American hospitals because of the costs of hospitalization. Therefore, heparin is given until revascularization is accomplished, or for 48 to 72 hours. The only time it would be administered longer (usually 96 to 120 hours) is if catheterization had shown clotting in the coronary arteries. There is some controversy as to whether ASA should be started immediately or delayed until heparin is stopped. Although data from Canada suggests that the combination of heparin and ASA increases the incidence of adverse bleeding events and adds no further reduction in cardiac events, most American physicians give both, as long as there are no contraindications to ASA usage. The dosage of ASA recommended in the guideline of 81 to 324 mg per day is quite a wide range. Most physicians either use 81 mg a day or the standard 324 mg per day, although there is a 160 mg ASA tablet available. Since there is no clear guideline as to which is best for preventing adverse events, the dose is usually based on the estimated tolerance of the patient to ASA. I tend to use 81 mg per day in patients with any history of ulcer or gastritis and in the elderly, whereas in younger patients with no history of such problems 324 mg per day is well tolerated, especially if it is enteric-coated. Although generic ASA tablets are inexpensive, I usually advise the patient to take a name brand, such as Bayer.

72 hours after symptom onset if serial CK and CK-MB (cardiac muscle) determinations are normal (strength of evidence = C).

Standard criteria for diagnosis of acute MI are based on demonstrating elevation and subsequent decline of CK levels along with evolutionary changes on serial 12-lead ECGs. CK is a nonstructural muscle enzyme that catalyzes the transfer of high energy phosphate from creatinine phosphate to adenosine diphosphate (ADP). CK occurs in three isoenzyme forms: skeletal muscle (MM), brain (BB), and MB (predominantly cardiac). CK-MB, the most sensitive and specific diagnostic test for acute MI, begins to rise within 6 hours of myocardial injury and peaks at 10 to 18 hours (Botker, Ravkilde, Sogaard et al., 1991). Total CK begins to rise at about 12 hours after symptom onset and peaks at 12 to 24 hours. Because of the rapid rise and clearance of CK-MB and total CK, timing of blood sampling is crucial in achieving maximal detection of acute MI. The literature is mixed, however, on the optimal sampling interval (Lee and Goldman, 1986). Rapid reporting of results of serial CK-MB measurements obtained hourly for 3 hours after presentation to the ED was found to aid early decision in 376 patients evaluated for chest pain (Young, Hedges, Gibler et al., 1991). After the admission sample, recommendations range from every 6 to every 12 hours for the first 24 hours. A sampling interval of every 6 to 8 hours is recommended to maximize sensitivity (Brush, Brand, Acampora et al., 1988).

Patients with severe renal insufficiency have a marked reduction in the clearance of CK from the blood. Diagnosis of acute MI in these patients is based not only on finding elevated CK and CK-MB levels but also demonstrating the rise and subsequent fall in these levels in relation to an appropriate clinical event. Patients presenting more than 24 hours after symptom onset who have negative serial CK-MBs should have serial LDH isoenzyme determinations. LDH is a widely distributed cellular enzyme that catalyzes the transformation of pyruvate to lactate. It has five isoenzymes identified on electrophoresis. LDH_1 is usually seen within 12 to 24 hours of myocardial necrosis and may fall to nondiagnostic levels by 72 hours.

Recently, several new laboratory tests for myocardial injury have been proposed with the goal of improving on the sensitivity and specificity of CK-MB. One such group of tests involves measuring the levels of CK-MM and -MB isoforms. Another group of tests concentrates on measuring serum levels of myocardial structural proteins, particularly troponin T, troponin I, myoglobin, and myosin light chain (Hamm, Ravkilde, Gerhardt et al., 1992; Katus, Yasuda, Gold et al., 1984). At present, none of these approaches has been established as providing more accurate diagnostic information than CK-MB. Thus, these tests are not currently recommended as part of standard practice.

The frequency of CK and CK-MB sampling has been the subject of several studies. A recent study compared CK-MB to troponin T and myoglobin in the assessment of possible MI. (deWinter et al., 1995) This study showed that although myoglobin was a good early marker of acute MI, it never reached the sensitivities and specificities of CK-MB. Troponin T achieved similar sensitivities and specificities as CK-MB, but only after 12 hours. CK-MB had the best sensitivity and specificity at approximately 12 hours. Thus, serial CK assays need to occur for at least 12 hours in order to ensure that the greatest sensitivity is exercised for detecting of myocardial ischemia. This is often accomplished by drawing a CK value on admission and then one at 8 hours and 16 hours later. Alternatively, one could truncate this and get a repeat sample at 6 and then 12 hours. The first value drawn may be useful if the patient has had pain for some time. If the value is normal, then a second sample can be taken 6 hours later. However, I think it is best for medico-legal purposes to take at least 2 samples over 12 hours before excluding an acute MI.

Recommendation: It is reasonable to measure serum lipid levels within 24 hours of admission unless patients have had a recent determination or are on chronic therapy for hyperlipidemia (strength of evidence = C). After 24 hours, determination of lipid levels should be deferred to the posthospital phase (strength of evidence = C).

Serum lipid levels (total cholesterol, triglycerides, high-density lipoprotein [HDL] cholesterol) provide an important part of the data base required for planning postdischarge management. Acute MI and other major physical stresses tend to falsely depress cholesterol and triglyceride levels, probably due to elevated circulating catecholamines. There are data, however, which show that cholesterol measured within the first 24 hours of an acute MI accurately reflects nonstress levels (Gore, Goldberg, Matsumoto et al., 1984). This is the rationale for the recommendation for an admission determination. All patients should also have a follow up determination no sooner than 8 weeks after their acute presentation (National Institutes of Health, 1990).

Recommendation: A followup ECG should be obtained 24 hours after admission and whenever the patient has recurrent symptoms or a change in clinical status (strength of evidence = C).

Serial ECGs are performed in unstable angina to detect the evolutionary changes of acute MI, transient and persistent ischemic complications, and disturbances of rhythm or conduction. In the absence of specific clinical indications, the optimal sampling interval for ECGs is uncertain. New data from continuous ST-segment monitoring show much more dynamic activity of the ST-segment in unstable angina patients than had been previously appreciated. Such patients may be in a tenuous equilibrium between coronary thrombus propagation and lysis with resulting intermittent transient coronary occlusion, often in the absence of symptoms. The therapeutic implication of these findings is still unclear. Also, continuous ST-segment monitoring is not widely available at present. Thus, the panel recommends that after the admission ECG, repeat ECGs should be obtained at 24 hours and then at 48 hours. In addition, a repeat ECG should be obtained whenever the patient's clinical condition changes (e.g., recurrent symptoms, hypotension, arrhythmia, pulmonary edema).

Recommendation: In patients who are hemodynamically stable, a portable chest radiograph should be obtained upon admission unless posteroanterior and lateral chest radiographs are likely to be obtained within 48 hours of admission. Chest radiographs should be obtained initially in all hemodynamically unstable patients and repeated as necessary to evaluate patients for pulmonary edema or for other specific indications (strength of evidence = C).

Because of lower cost and greater diagnostic content, a posteroanterior and lateral chest radiograph is preferable to a portable radiograph in patients with unstable angina who are hemodynamically stable. In general the chest radiograph does not contribute substantially to the initial management of these patients and, therefore, is reasonable to defer until other more pressing management concerns have been addressed. However, any suggestion of hemodynamic instability or inclusion of an alternative diagnosis of severe intrathoracic disease is reason for an early chest radiograph, even if it must be obtained by a portable technique.

Recommendation: In patients who do not undergo early cardiac catheterization but who have had evidence of ischemia, previous infarction, or conduction abnormalities on their resting ECG or have cardiomegaly by physical examination or chest radiograph, resting LV function should be assessed within 72 hours of admission using either a radionuclide ventriculogram or a two-dimensional echocardiogram (strength of evidence = C).

The resting EF is one of the most potent prognostic factors in CAD. In patients who are planned for early cardiac catheterization, this measurement can be obtained by contrast ventriculography. Clinicians who opt for an early conservative strategy (defined in Chapter 7) should obtain a resting noninvasive measure of LV function within 72 hours of admission in patients with previous infarction or cardiomegaly on chest radiograph to allow for additional risk stratification and identification of high-risk patients who should be referred for early angiography. Patients with low EFs (<0.50) should receive careful consideration for revascularization therapy because of the risk with medical therapy that increases as a function of decrease in EF. Selection of the imaging mode should be based primarily on the technology and expertise available at each site. Calculation of the EF using 2-D echocardiography is technically more difficult than by radionuclide ventriculography because of the cross-sectional nature of the images and the frequency of suboptimal sound penetration of the chest wall.

Assessment of Efficacy of Initial Medical Therapy

Recommendation: After patients are hemodynamically stable on an appropriate initial medical regimen, consideration should be given to early invasive management (strength of evidence = A).

An early management strategy characterized by cardiac catheterization within 48 hours of presentation for high-risk unstable angina, with consideration of subsequent revascularization by PTCA or CABG, has been shown by the TIMI IIIB trial (1994) to provide equivalent freedom from cardiac death but better pain relief than a conservative strategy that utilizes interventional approaches only with documented failure of a medical regimen (evidence cited in Chapter 7). A more complete discussion of factors likely to influence choice of these alternate approaches for an individual patient appears in Chapter 7.

LV function should be assessed as early as possible after admission, in order to choose the most appropriate pharmacologic therapy for the patient beyond ASA, heparin, and NTG. We usually recommend echocardiography rather than radionuclide angiography for several reasons. First, it can be done at the bedside, if necessary, without moving the patient to a laboratory. Second, considerably more information is obtained about the patient's heart, and finally, it is less expensive in most hospitals. About 5 percent of patients will have an inadequate echo study for the assessment of LV function. In these patients, a radionuclide angiogram can be considered. Delaying echocardiography until the catheterization is done, so that the left ventriculogram can be substituted, is not a good practice. If the echocardiogram is of good quality, then there is no need to perform an LV angiogram during the cardiac catheterization. This decreases the dye load and the time that catheters are in the body. Obviously, if the catheterization is performed early and LV arteriography is done, then there is no need for an echocardiogram to assess LV function, unless the angiogram is technically inadequate.

Patient counseling to provide information, discuss relative risks and benefits, and learn patient preference about further treatment with the early invasive or conservative strategies is appropriate after the patient has reached a plateau of stabilization. This important counseling period should be scheduled for a time permitting medical practitioners to completely address these serious issues with several brief intervals of groups discussion separated by periods of private reflection for the patient and family and/or advocate. In this elective setting, patients should not be hurried into making this major decision. Patients who choose an early invasive strategy will be managed as described in Chapter 7. The remaining patients will continue to be treated with a medical regimen appropriate for the severity of symptoms and will retain the option for invasive therapy if medical therapy proves ineffective.

Recommendation: The goal of medical therapy for unstable angina is to institute a regimen in which patients receive daily ASA (160 to 324 mg) and IV heparin (adjusted to maintain an aPTT value of 1.5 to 2.5 times control) plus nitrates and beta blockers (with a resting heart rate ≤60 beats/min). Calcium channel blockers may be added in the subset of patients with significant hypertension (SBP >150 mmHg), in patients who have refractory ischemia on beta blockers, and in patients with variant angina. Recurrent symptoms after the initial hemodynamic goals of therapy have been achieved may be re-

garded as a failure of medical therapy and should prompt consideration of urgent cardiac catheterization (strength of evidence = C).

Patients who desire a noninterventional strategy of early treatment of unstable angina will be started on an initial medical regimen with serial reassessments to determine the success of therapy and the occurrence of significant complications. During the initial hours of therapy, medications are titrated up to their target doses as permitted by the patient's hemodynamic state and general medical condition. Prior to achievement of the target regimen, the patient may have recurrent symptoms requiring the physician to consider whether a change in course (such as emergency catheterization) would be appropriate. In addition, once the desired level of medical therapy has been reached, recurrent symptoms may indicate a need for a still more intensive regimen or for triage to early cardiac catheterization. Thus, clinical decisionmaking at this juncture requires criteria by which the adequacy of medical therapy can be judged and failure of such therapy defined. In addition, it is necessary to understand the prognostic importance of the different manifestations of recurrent ischemia so that changes in management can be formulated based on the patient's short-term risk of adverse events.

Criteria defining the adequacy of medical therapy in unstable angina serve two roles: first, they provide the practitioner with explicit therapeutic goals to ensure that patients receive the full benefits available from such therapies; and second, they provide guidance about the conditions under which early diagnostic catheterization and subsequent revascularization should be considered. If inadequate levels of medical therapy are employed, recurrent symptoms may precipitate an otherwise avoidable referral for invasive study. On the other hand, excessively aggressive therapeutic endpoints may provoke harmful complications or needlessly delay revascularization in patients likely to benefit from this therapy.

The optimal level of medical therapy for the unstable angina patient has not yet been established. Two general approaches have been proposed to define adequate medical therapy. The first defines adequate medical therapy as maximally tolerated doses of nitrates, beta blockers, and calcium channel blockers plus ASA and heparin. The implication of this definition is that failure of medical therapy cannot be declared until each drug has been pushed up to limiting levels so that any further increment would cause hemodynamic deterioration or toxicity. The second approach is to define adequate medical therapy by arbitrary levels of each of the key therapeutic agents. For example, in addition to heparin and ASA, this criterion might require the patient to be on IV nitrates (e.g., ≥ 50 µg/min) or nonparenteral nitrates (e.g., ≥ 1 inch of ointment) and a combination of beta blockers and calcium channel blockers with a heart rate ≤ 60 beats per minute and an SBP ≤ 150 mmHg. Since achievement of steady state medication effects may require 24 hours or more even with parenteral administration, some criteria for adequate medical therapy also specify a minimum duration such therapy should be continued prior to referral for invasive study. Intensive medical treatment for unstable angina is usually very effective. In one recent study, only 11 of 502 patients (2%) admitted for unstable angina were found to be truly refractory to medical therapy (Grambow and Topol, 1992).

Based on current understanding of the most prevalent pathophysiology of unstable angina (i.e., plaque rupture with thrombus formation and propagation), it is proposed that failure of medical therapy be defined in terms of continuing angina despite having an adequate anticoagulant effect with at least moderate reductions in cardiac oxygen demand through decreases in heart rate and blood pressure. Thus, for this guideline a patient will not be said to have failed (or be "refractory" to) medical therapy until he or she is receiving ASA (≥160 mg/day) and IV heparin with an aPTT of 1.5 to 2.5 times control. In addition, in the absence of limiting symptoms, IV NTG should be infused at ≥50 µg/min (or topical NTG at ≥1 inch of ointment every 6 hours for three doses followed by a 6- to 8-hour nitrate-free interval or an equivalent regimen of oral or buccal nitrates). Beta blockers should be used to keep the resting heart rate at an average of ≤60 beats/minute. Significant hypertension (i.e., resting SBP ≥150 mmHg) resistant to first-line medical therapy is an indication for addition of calcium channel blockers.

Although it is theoretically desirable to have this regimen in place for ≥24 hours before declaring any patient a failure of medical therapy, to do so in all cases may be inappropriate or even dangerous. In particular, patients who have one or more recurrent severe, prolonged (>20 minutes) ischemic episodes particularly when accompanied by pulmonary edema, a new or worsening MR murmur, hypotension, or new ST- or T-wave changes should be considered high risk, regardless of the level of medical therapy, and triaged to early cardiac catheterization. Patients with shorter, less severe ischemic episodes without accompanying hemodynamic or ECG changes are at substantially lower risk and should be continued on medical therapy to the prespecified targets.

Evaluation and Management of Early Ischemic Complications

The major ischemic complications seen in unstable angina are acute MI, recurrent unstable angina, acute ischemic pulmonary edema, new or worsening MR, cardiogenic shock, malignant ventricular arrhythmias, and advanced AV block. Aside from maximizing the medical regimen described in the previous section and instituting appropriate adjunctive therapy (e.g., pulmonary artery pressure monitoring and inotropic therapy for shock, antiarrhythmic therapy for malignant ventricular arrhythmias, pacemaker for symptomatic high-grade AV block), the clinician should consider either insertion of an IABP or cardiac catheterization or both.

Intra-aortic Balloon Pumping.

Recommendation: An IABP should be considered in unstable angina patients

Since most patients stabilize on intensified medical treatment, the major issue in this phase is weaning the patient off IV medications and on to oral ones. If a patient is pain-free after 24 hours of IV NTG, it is usually tapered over 3 hours. If a patient has known coronary disease, another form of oral or topical nitrates may be substituted for IV at this time. For the patient in whom a diagnosis of coronary disease is uncertain, it is often best to observe the patient off IV nitrates to see if any episodes of chest pain occur, and if so, to try to get ECGs during these episodes. IV heparin is usually continued if the patient is going to catheterization, but if noninvasive testing has been chosen, then the IV heparin is often stopped as well. Naturally, the patients are kept on ASA and any other antianginal medicines they are taking, unless they are believed to be inappropriate at this time.

It would be ideal to stop all antianginal medications prior to stress testing in patients without known CAD, but this is often not possible in practice. It has been shown that antianginal medications will reduce the number of true-positive exercise tests, running the risk of missing significant disease in a chest pain patient. On the other hand, some patients cannot be taken off medications because symptoms may return or an event may occur. Also, the demonstration of myocardial ischemia on medical therapy is important information suggesting that an invasive approach is required. Thus, only in patients with a low risk of events would discontinuation of antianginal medications be considered.

who have symptoms refractory to aggressive medical management or hemodynamic instability if emergency cardiac catheterization is not possible or as a bridge to stabilize the patient on the way to the catheterization laboratory or the operating room (strength of evidence = B). Exceptions to this recommendation are made for patients with severe peripheral vascular disease, significant aortic insufficiency, or known severe aorto-iliac disease including aortic aneurysm (strength of evidence = C). Placement of an IABP for stabilization may precede or follow diagnostic catheterization depending on specific circumstances, such as the anticipated delay for alternate approaches and level of expertise available in the immediate care environment (strength of evidence = C).

Recommendation: Patients not stabilized after placement of an IABP should be re-evaluated to ensure proper functioning of the device and to reaffirm that the most likely diagnosis remains unstable angina. If so, consideration should be given to emergency catheterization (strength of evidence = B).

IABP counterpulsation is a method of providing temporary circulatory assistance in the form of reduced afterload and increased coronary perfusion pressure. The balloon catheter is placed percutaneously via the femoral artery and positioned in the descending thoracic aorta with the tip of the catheter several centimeters distal to the left subclavian artery. The device is synchronized with the ECG or arterial pulse tracing so that the balloon is rapidly inflated during diastole (after closure of the aortic valve) with an inert gas (helium) and rapidly deflated just before the onset of systole (and opening of the aortic valve). The IABP produces a significant reduction in afterload with a consequent reduction in myocardial work and oxygen demand. It also increases the cardiac output by a modest amount (usually 10 to 20%, depending on the extent of LV dysfunction). Finally, the IABP increases thoracic aortic diastolic pressure with a consequent increase in coronary perfusion pressure. Whether this latter effect increases coronary blood flow distal to a critical coronary stenosis or decreases the likelihood of early progression to complete coronary occlusion remains controversial.

Consecutive series of patients admitted to the hospital for unstable angina show the IABP to be required for symptom control in only about 1 percent of cases (White, Lee, and Cook, 1990). Because patients entering the initial intensive management phase represent the highest risk subgroup of patients with unstable angina, the need for IABP in this subgroup is anticipated to be in the range of 3 percent. The IABP almost always stabilizes patients with severe myocardial ischemia and causes an almost immediate and dramatic relief of pain and ECG changes (Rankin, Newton, Califf et al., 1984). Therefore, the persistence of continued symptoms after introduction of the IABP suggests that unstable angina is not the total etiology of the presenting condition, and further evaluation should be pursued as mandated by signs or symptoms of other primary or associated disorders. Reassessment should be made for other potentially devastating causes of symptoms that could be mistaken for unstable angina, such as pneumothorax, aortic dissection, dissecting aneurysm, esophageal rupture, or perforated peptic ulcer.

There are no randomized trials of IABP use in unstable angina. Uncontrolled series suggest that it is a very effective short-term method of stabilizing the unstable angina patient (Aroesty, Weintraub, Paulin et al., 1979). In experienced centers, approximately 10 to 15 percent of patients will develop vascular complications with prolonged use of balloon pumps, often compromising distal limb blood flow (Kantrowitz, Wasfie, Freed et al., 1986; Makhoul, Cole, and McCann, 1993). For this reason, patients receiving an IABP should be maintained on full-dose IV heparin with serial monitoring of aPTT, unless contraindications to heparin therapy exist. About half of ischemic leg complications are reversed by pump removal; many of the remainder require an embolectomy procedure.

In summary, experience shows that use of an IABP can be a very effective temporizing measure to allow stabilization of high-risk acute unstable angina patients. However, no clinical trials have established the optimal parameters for this inter-

IABP placement should never be done unless there is a definitive plan for the patient and a set length of time for which balloon pumping will be performed. IABP is highly effective at maintaining circulatory adequacy and relieving unstable angina in patients with severe coronary disease. Unless a definite plan is made, patients can become balloon-dependent and decisions on withdrawing balloon support can be very difficult. The reason we do not have "Do Not Balloon" orders, like we have "Do Not Intubate" or "Do Not Resuscitate," is because cardiologists have been very careful to put balloon pumps only in patients for which they have a definite plan and for whom there is set time limit on the balloon's use. Usually, after IABP, the patient is taken to the catheterization laboratory and it is determined if there is anything that can be corrected by revascularization or other forms of intervention or surgery. If nothing is found, either the balloon is removed or the balloon is used for 48 to 72 hours while medical therapy is intensified. This gives adequate time for patients with whom there is no revascularization possible to improve their intrinsic cardiac state. It also gives time to stabilize other medical conditions that may be exacerbating or exaggerating their ischemic heart disease problem.

vention. Because of the complications associated with use of this procedure, it should be attempted only in centers that have clinicians experienced in the placement of the device and have access to emergency vascular surgery support should it be required.

Emergency/Urgent Cardiac Catheterization.

Recommendation: If chest discomfort with objective evidence of ischemia persists for ≥1 hour after aggressive medical therapy, triage to emergency cardiac catheterization should be strongly considered (strength of evidence = B).

Recommendation: Urgent cardiac catheterization should be considered in patients with unstable angina who have recurrent ischemic episodes despite appropriate medical therapy or who have high-risk unstable angina (strength of evidence = B).

Recommendation: Acute revascularization is indicated for patients with refractory pain (≥1 hour on aggressive medical therapy) who are found at catheterization to have an acutely occluded major coronary vessel, or severe subtotal occlusion of a culprit vessel, or severe multivessel disease with impaired LV function (strength of evidence = B).

In this guideline, emergency catheterization refers to a diagnostic catheterization study that is performed immediately or as soon as possible (i.e., <6 hours) after the precipitating event. Urgent catheterization is performed because of less severe precipitating events or because the patient exhibits features of high-risk unstable angina (see Table 9). Urgent catheterization is usually performed within 24 hours of presentation of the precipitating event. Elective catheterization, which is discussed in Chapter 7, is used to describe all diagnostic catheterization procedures not meeting the above criteria.

Since cardiac catheterization is a diagnostic procedure, it provides health benefits only when it yields information that can be used to plan and execute effective therapies. Thus, the utility of catheterization is tied closely to the subsequent decisions about triage for revascularization. Evidence for benefit of revascularization based on cardiac catheterization findings is discussed in Chapter 7. Unstable angina patients meeting criteria for emergency catheterization commonly have at least one of the following findings:

1. An apparently recent coronary occlusion with absent or very slow flow (TIMI perfusion grades 0 or 1),[2] which can present without diagnostic ST-segment elevation most commonly in the setting of a left circumflex (or branch) occlusion.
2. A critical stenosis (≥95%) of the left main coronary artery or a major coronary vessel.
3. Severe multivessel disease.
4. Severe aortic outflow tract obstruction, usually due to severe aortic stenosis, with coexisting significant CAD.

Because of the high-risk nature of this population, options for emergency surgical referral should be clearly defined prior to initiation of the catheterization procedure.

Patients found at catheterization to have an occluded culprit vessel (defined as the vessel most likely by location and angiographic appearance to be responsible for the observed ischemia) and ongoing pain/ischemia with a total symptom duration of >12 hours should in most cases undergo emergency revascularization. This may take the form of primary PTCA, intracoronary thrombolytic therapy with adjunctive PTCA as necessary, or emergency bypass surgery. Because the risks of PTCA are increased in the setting of an acutely unstable plaque relative to stable CAD, the strategy for acute intervention has often been to do only as much as necessary to restore adequate distal flow and relieve symptoms but no more. In some cases, repeat coronary contrast injections, with or without intracoronary thrombolytic therapy, may confirm improvement in distal flow so that acute revascular-

---

[2]Perfusion grade=0 indicates no antegrade flow beyond the occlusion. Perfusion grade=1 indicates penetration without perfusion where the contrast material passes beyond the obstruction but "hangs up" and does not opacify the entire coronary bed distal to the obstruction (TIMI Study Group, 1985).

ization is not necessary. In these patients, placement of an IABP plus continuation of IV heparin may allow further intervention to be deferred for several days when it can be performed under more controlled, more elective circumstances with lower risk of abrupt closure or other complications. However, timing of PTCA in this setting remains controversial.

Data on the effects of acute catheterization on death and nonfatal MI come from the TIMI IIIB study (TIMI IIIB, 1994), which showed that at 42 days early invasive and early conservative strategies were associated with equivalent "hard" outcomes of death and MI (discussed in detail in Chapter 7). In addition, the early invasive strategy showed a reduction in late recurrent ischemia, use of antianginal medication, and need for rehospitalization.

Patients with persistent ischemia who do not have adequate distal flow established after initial contrast injections and who are not candidates for PTCA, for example because of severe three-vessel or left main disease, should be considered for emergency placement of an IABP. Consultation with a cardiac surgeon about the options for triage to emergency CABG surgery for these patients should take place as soon as possible.

Preparation for Nonintensive Phase

Recommendation: Patients who become asymptomatic should be progressively mobilized and instructed to notify their health care team if mobilization causes recurrent symptoms (strength of evidence = C).

Recommendation: If parenteral nitrate and beta-blocker therapy was required initially, such regimens can be converted to nonparenteral regimens after the patient has been stable and pain free for at least 24 hours (strength of evidence = C).

The large majority of unstable angina patients will stabilize and become pain-free with appropriate intensive medical therapy. Transfer from intensive to nonintensive medical management is undertaken when the patient is hemodynamically stable (including no uncompensated CHF) and ischemia has been successfully suppressed for ≥24 hours. Once these criteria are satisfied, any parenteral medicines can be converted to nonparenteral regimens in preparation for this transfer. Heparin use should be reassessed after 24 hours and may be discontinued in selected patients, such as those who are found to have a clearly identified secondary cause for unstable angina (e.g., anemia). ASA is continued without interruption.

Patient Counseling

Recommendation: Life situation, anxiety-level, and coping skills should be assessed and support offered by the health care team. Patients who continue to have high levels of anxiety should be given anxiolytic agents as needed (strength of evidence = C).

In most cases, the first option for relieving anxiety should be counseling by the health care team. Patients should be encouraged to discuss their life situation and knowledge and concerns about the import of their disease on their life. Orientation of the patient to the unit, its routines, and the type of care they are likely to receive often allays needless fears. Counseling about diagnostic and treatment alternatives should continue in as positive a tone as permitted by the severity of the situation. For some patients, speaking with a member of the clergy may provide additional reassurance. If these strategies are ineffective, judicious use of an anxiolytic agent may assist in decreasing sympathetic tone and resulting ischemia.

Recomendation: Counseling should continue in this phase regarding the significance of clinical events that have occurred and management alternatives. Where appropriate, the health care team should reassure the patient that a functional recovery is possible and indicate how soon the patient may be able to resume his or her activities (strength of evidence = C).

As the health care team prepares to move the patient into the nonintensive medical management phase, it is often a good time to reiterate for the patient the significance of events that have taken place during the period of intense medical management. The slower pace of events and less intensive care at the conclusion of this phase affords the patient some time to adjust to his or her condition and hospitalization.

Conclusion of Intensive Medical Management Phase

Patients with unstable angina whose symptoms are controlled for ≥24 hours with intensive medical therapy should be stratified according to whether the diagnosis of acute MI or no MI has been made. Patients with unstable angina, as well as those with non-Q-wave MI who remain free of symptoms or signs of ischemia, should appropriately pass to the nonintensive hospital management phase. Patients with persisting symptomatic unstable angina during the first 24 hours will be advised to undergo cardiac catheterization and myocardial revascularization if the anatomy is suitable and if they have no contraindications. Patients who prefer continued intensive medical management to cardiac catheterization and myocardial revascularization or are not candidates for these procedures will continue to receive intensive care at a level and for a duration dictated by the level of their disease activity.

Medical Record

The medical record should include or update the following minimal information in addition to the information available on admission:

- Diagnosis established (unstable angina, non-Q-wave MI, Q-wave MI).
- The intensity of pain (1 to 10) and duration (<20 minutes, <1 hour, >1 hour) of each episode of angina or equivalent ischemic symptoms.

- The duration of the longest anginal episode during the phase.
- Major or minor complications of diagnosis or treatment during this phase.
- Summary of pharmacologic therapy used.
- Documentation of the status of patient teaching including evidence of what the patient appears to understand.
- Documentation of alternate treatment options discussed with the patient.
- Deaths classified as noncardiac or cardiac.
- Cardiac deaths classified as precipitated by arrhythmia, progressive ischemia, or progressive cardiac failure.

Duration of Intensive Medical Management Phase

Typically, most high-risk, unstable angina patients can be stabilized within 24 to 48 hours of admission to the ICU. Some unstable patients will progress to sustain a transmural MI and others will require urgent cardiac catheterization, PTCA, or CABG. However, the majority of patients will rapidly become asymptomatic on aggressive medical therapy. Patients who remain asymptomatic for 24 hours may be transferred to a regular hospital room for initiation of the nonintensive phase of management.

5

Guideline: Progression to Nonintensive Medical Management

Commentary by Michael H. Crawford, M.D.

Introduction

High-risk and some intermediate-risk unstable angina patients will be moved to the nonintensive phase after 1 or more days of intensive management and stabilization. Some of these latter patients will have undergone cardiac catheterization, and some also will have had one or more revascularization procedures. Other intermediate-risk unstable angina patients may be admitted initially to a monitored intermediate care unit until the diagnosis of MI can be excluded and it is clear that the patient's symptoms are adequately controlled on medical therapy. These patients then enter the nonintensive phase of management. Still other intermediate-risk and some low-risk patients may be admitted directly to a regular hospital bed with telemetry capabilities, thereby proceeding directly to the nonintensive phase. Management of the nonintensive phase is described in this chapter (see Figure 8).

Objectives of Care

Transfer out of the intensive care phase is an important indicator that the patient has progressed to a lower risk state. At this point, emphasis shifts from acute stabilization to design of a maintenance medical regimen that will suppress reactivation of acute disease activity. In addition, a major focus is placed on risk stratification with primary goals of assessing the future risk of adverse cardiac events, the sufficiency of medical therapy in controlling symptoms, and the need for diagnostic cardiac catheterization and revascularization. Use of noninvasive testing is detailed in Chapter 6, and indications for catheterization and revascularization are described in Chapter 7. This chapter will describe the general care of patients who have reached the nonintensive phase of care. By this point in the hospital course, most patients with acute MI have been identified; their subsequent management is outside the scope of this guideline.

Approach to Care Objectives

Once patients reach the nonintensive phase of management, reasons for continued hospitalization include optimization of medical therapy, evaluation of the propensity for recurrent ischemia or ischemic complications, and risk stratification to determine the need for catheterization and revascularization. Continuous monitoring of the ECG at this phase is generally unnecessary. All patients should be instructed to notify nursing personnel immediately if chest discomfort recurs. Recurrent ischemic episodes should prompt a brief nursing assessment and an emergent ECG and generally should be brought to the attention of a physician. The patient's medical regimen should be re-evaluated and doses of anti-ischemic agents should be increased as tolerated. Patients who have pain or ECG evidence of ischemia increasing in severity for >20 minutes and unresponsive to NTG should be transferred to the intensive management phase protocol. Patients who respond to sublingual NTG do not need to be transferred. However, a second recurrence of chest pain of at least 20 minutes duration in the setting of appropriate medical therapy should prompt return of the patient to a monitored environment and the management steps outlined in the intensive management phase.

In general, patients reaching this phase would be referred within 1 to 2 days either for noninvasive functional testing or for cardiac catheterization. Selection of the appropriate strategy of risk stratification is discussed in Chapters 6 and 7. Patients can be considered ready for discharge from the hospital when their evaluation is complete and an appropriate outpatient therapeutic regimen is established.

Patient Counseling

Recommendation: During this phase, the patient should gradually progress under the observation of the health care team to a level of activity commensurate with the amount of activity required to perform activities of daily living (strength of evidence = C).

Recommendation: In this phase, the patient and his or her family should begin to work toward risk-factor modification goals (strength of evidence = C).

Steps to move the patient towards readiness for hospital discharge should be initiated during this phase. These steps include instruction on home diet and exercise, physical activity, resumption of sexual relations, return to work, and resumption of driving and other usual activities. In addition, detailed discussions should be conducted with the patient, his or her family, and the patient's advocate to review the events since presentation and their significance, current status, diagnostic and therapeutic options, and general prognosis.

The slower pace of this phase of the patient's hospitalization, in contrast to early stabilization and intensive care, offers the most appropriate time for CAD edu-

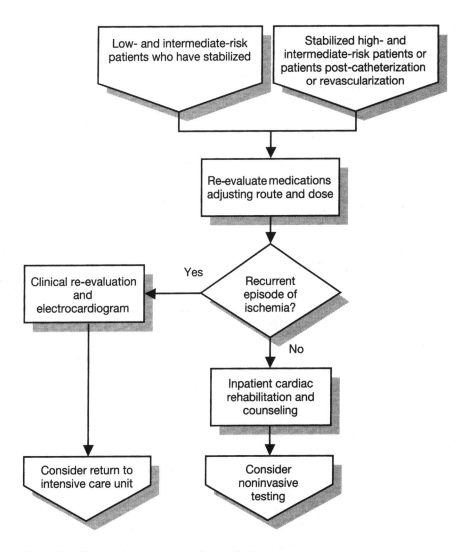

Figure 8.   Progression to nonintensive medical management.

Once patients are off IV medications they can be moved to a less intensive care unit, which may be a cardiac subacute unit or a regular ward. At this point, if the patients have no arrhythmias, ECG monitoring is not necessary, but is often done for an additional 24 hours, if the capability exists, just to make sure that the stress of transfer to a new environment does not precipitate any rhythm disturbances. If a noninvasive evaluation approach has been chosen, it should be completed as quickly as possible, so that the patient can be discharged if he or she is deemed to be at low risk for a cardiac event.

cation. During the initial phase of the hospitalization, the patient may be in much pain, under sedation, or generally too anxious to retain the information. Likewise, immediately before discharge the patient may be distracted by preparations for going home.

Medical Record

The following information should be added to the medical record during this phase of care:

■ Medications at the beginning and conclusion of this phase of care.
■ The number, severity, and duration of ischemic episodes.
■ Complications occurring during this phase.
■ Evaluation of the patient's understanding of recommended lifestyle changes and an assessment of the patient's willingness to adhere to recommendations.

Duration of Nonintensive Medical Management Phase

The nonintensive phase of management begins with ICU or intermediate care unit transfer and extends until hospital discharge. During this phase, risk stratification will be completed, and many patients will undergo cardiac catheterization and revascularization procedures. Thus, low-risk patients not requiring further intervention may be discharged in 1 to 2 days, but patients with complicated cases or those requiring CABG may require an additional week or more of hospitalization.

6

Guideline: Noninvasive Testing

Commentary by Michael H. Crawford, M.D.

Background

The entire process of managing patients with unstable angina requires ongoing risk stratification. Much prognostic information of value derives from the initial assessment and the patient's subsequent course over the first few days of management, as described in Chapters 3 and 4. In many cases, noninvasive stress testing provides a useful supplement to these clinically based risk assessments.

However, some patients, such as those with rest angina and ECG-documented ischemia, have such a high likelihood of CAD and risk of adverse events that noninvasive risk stratification would not be likely to identify a subgroup with sufficiently low risk to merit noninterventional strategies. Other patients are not willing to consider interventional treatment or have severe complicating illnesses or advanced age so that referral for revascularization would not be reasonable. Still other patients may be felt to have a very low likelihood of CAD after their initial complete clinical evaluation with an associated risk of cardiac events so low that no positive test finding would prompt consideration of catheterization and myocardial revascularization. All patients who do not fall into one of the above exception categories are reasonable candidates for risk stratification by noninvasive testing (see Figure 9).

Objectives of Care

The goals of noninvasive testing in a patient with unstable angina who has recently been stabilized are to estimate the subsequent prognosis, especially for the next 3 to 6 months, to decide what additional tests and adjustments in therapy are required based on this prognosis, and to provide the patient with the information and reassurances necessary to return to a lifestyle as full and productive as possible.

Approach to Care Objectives

Selection of Noninvasive Tests

Recommendation: Exercise or pharmacologic stress testing should generally be an integral part of the outpatient evaluation of low-risk patients with unstable angina. In most cases, testing should be done within 72 hours of presentation (strength of evidence = B).

Recommendation: Unless cardiac catheterization is indicated, noninvasive exercise or pharmacologic stress testing should be performed in low- or intermediate-risk patients (see Table 8) hospitalized with unstable angina who have been free of angina and CHF for a minimum of 48 hours (strength of evidence = B).

Recommendation: Choice of initial stress testing modality should be based on an evaluation of the patient's resting ECG, his or her physical ability to perform exercise, and the local expertise and technologies available. In general, the exercise treadmill test should be the standard mode of stress testing employed in patients with a normal ECG who are not taking digoxin. Patients with widespread resting ST depression (≥1 mm), ST changes secondary to digoxin, LV hypertrophy, LBBB/significant intraventricular conduction deficit (IVCD), or pre-excitation usually should be tested using an imaging modality. Patients unable to exercise due to physical limitations (e.g., arthritis, amputation, severe peripheral vascular disease [PVD], severe COPD, general debility) should undergo pharmacologic stress testing in combination with an imaging modality (strength of evidence = B).

Recommendation: Choice among the different imaging modalities that can be used with exercise or pharmacologic stress testing should be based primarily on the local expertise available to perform and interpret the study (strength of evidence = C).

Noninvasive functional or stress testing refers to a series of provocative tests that use either exercise or pharmacologic means to detect ischemia or inhomogeneity in myocardial blood flow due to obstructive CAD. The exercise tests are based on the principle of using a progressive physiologic stress (usually treadmill or bicycle exercise) to increase myocardial work and oxygen demand while using some method (ECG, function, perfusion) to document objective evidence of ischemia. Provocation of ischemia at a low workload (e.g., <5 to 6 metabolic equivalents [METs]) signifies a high-risk patient who would generally merit referral to cardiac catheterization. On the other hand, attainment of a higher workload (e.g., ≥5 to 6 METs) without ischemia is associated with a better prognosis, and many such patients can be safely managed conservatively. Other patients, including

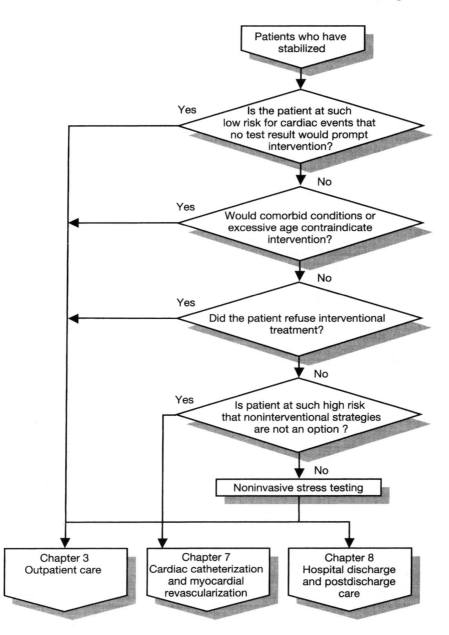

Figure 9. Patient flow: Noninvasive testing.

those who tolerate only a low workload but have no evident ischemia or those who develop ischemia at a high workload, represent an intermediate-risk group for whom several reasonable strategies can be proposed.

Pharmacologic stress testing provides an important complement to exercise testing, particularly for the subset of patients who are unable to exercise (Zhu, Chung, Botvinick et al., 1991). The IV-administered coronary vasodilators such as dipyridamole decrease coronary vascular resistance and thus substantially increase coronary flow. Where significant epicardial coronary stenosis exists, the increase in flow is limited relative to myocardial segments supplied by nonobstructed coronary arteries. This flow discrepancy is routinely evaluated with perfusion scintigraphy. Occasionally, these agents produce ischemia by provoking an endocardial to epicardial steal and consequent diminished endocardial blood flow in the territory of a critical coronary stenosis. In contrast, dobutamine stress testing with measurement of cardiac function or perfusion acts by increasing myocardial oxygen demand in a fashion similar to exercise.

The greatest experience with these agents is in patients who are unable to exercise. In general, their prognostic value appears equivalent to exercise testing with imaging although there are few direct comparison studies of prognostic stratification with the two approaches. However, the known prognostic information derived from maximal exercise level attained argues for use of pharmacologic stress testing as an alternative to exercise testing only for specific indications.

No empirical data or theoretical arguments have yet established that LV function during exercise or pharmacologic stress provides more valuable prognostic information than a perfusion scan or vice versa. Both the extent of CAD and the degree of LV dysfunction are important for selection of appropriate therapy. Studies directly comparing prognostic information from multiple noninvasive tests for ischemia in patients after stabilization of unstable angina are hampered by small sample size (Amanullah, Bevegard, Lindvall et al., 1992; Marmur, Freeman, Langer et al., 1990).

Two relatively large studies addressed the prognostic value of exercise testing in unstable angina to predict death and MI. The Multicenter Myocardial Ischemia Research Group recently reported the results of a 23-month followup study of the prognostic value of noninvasive testing in 936 stable CAD patients who had an MI (70%) or unstable angina (30%) hospitalization within the 6-month period prior to testing (Moss, Goldstein, Hall et al., 1993). Noninvasive testing involved rest, ambulatory, and exercise ECG and stress thallium-201 scintigraphy. The outcome event tested was a composite of death (n = 22), nonfatal MI (n = 53), or unstable angina (n = 125). In the primary analysis, only ST depression on the resting ECG was an independent prognostic factor. Both exercise ECG ST depression (p = 0.29) and reversible thallium defects (p = 0.05) showed univariate trends towards a worse prognosis. Ambulatory ECG changes were not significant predictors of outcome in this population (p = 0.93). Additional prespecified analyses revealed that the combination of exercise ST depression >0.10 mV and an exercise duration <9 minutes (modified Bruce protocol) identified patients at a 3.4-fold (<6 minutes) to 1.9-fold (6 to 9 minutes) increase in risk of cardiac events. With the exercise thallium, a reversible defect and increased lung thallium uptake indicated a 2.8-fold increase in risk; a reversible defect alone signified a 1.2-fold increase in risk.

The RISC study group evaluated the use of predischarge symptom-limited, bicycle exercise testing in 740 men admitted with unstable angina (51%) or non-Q-wave MI (49%) (Nyman, Larsson, Areskog et al., 1992). Multivariate analysis showed that the extent of ischemic ST depression (number of positive leads) and low maximal workload were independent predictors of 1-year, infarct-free survival.

In addition to these two large studies, 6 studies of patients with unstable angina report at least 10 cardiac deaths and/or MIs during followup (see Table 16). These studies permit comparison of the effectiveness of exercise ECG and exercise or dipyridamole thallium-201 for risk stratification. The total annualized risk of cardiac events in each study is depicted in Figure 10, with the individual studies arranged from left to right in ascending order of risk. This arrangement places studies in populations at lower risk on the left and at higher risk of subsequent event on the right. The annualized percentage risk in the high- and low-risk groups stratified by a positive or negative noninvasive test is plotted using criteria defined as optimal for each study. All three studies show similar accuracy in dichotomizing the total population into low- and high-risk subgroups.

In low-risk patients, it is unclear that an imaging modality adds importantly to a standard treadmill test. Thus, selection of the test to use with an individual patient should rest primarily on patient characteristics, knowledge of local availability, and interpretation expertise. Because of simplicity, lower cost, and widespread familiarity with performance and interpretation, the standard ECG treadmill is the most reasonable test to select in patients able to exercise who have a normal resting ECG. Patients with an abnormal baseline ECG that would interfere with interpretation of the exercise results should have an imaging modality added to their test. Patients unable to exercise should have a pharmacologic stress test. The optimal testing strategy in women remains less well-defined than in men. All major forms of exercise testing have been reported as less accurate for diagnosis in women. At least a portion of the lower reported accuracy derives from a lower pretest likelihood of CAD in populations of women compared with men. The relative accuracy of noninvasive testing for prognosis in women and men has not been adequately studied. Until data are reported to clarify this issue, it is reasonable to use noninvasive testing for prognosis in women as freely as in men with proper consideration of the influence of sex on the pretest likelihood of CAD.

The stress test using a standard protocol can be performed as soon as appropriate indications are present and the patient has stabilized clinically. In 1991, Larsson, Areskog, Areskog and colleagues compared the results of a symptom-limited exercise test performed before discharge at 3 to 7 days after an episode of

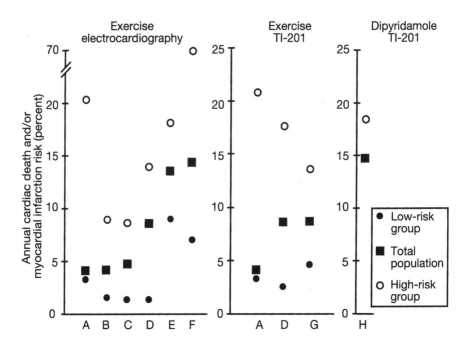

Figure 10.   Noninvasive testing for risk stratification in patients with unstable angina. **Source:** Studies summarized in Table 10.

unstable angina or non-Q-wave infarction with the results of a similar test 1 month later in 189 patients. The diagnostic and prognostic value of both tests was similar, but the earlier test identified events occurring over the first month which represented one-half of all events during the first year. This study illustrates the importance of early noninvasive testing for risk stratification of patients with unstable angina.

Use of Noninvasive Test Results in Patient Management

Recommendation: Patients with a low-risk exercise test result (predicted average annual cardiac mortality <1%/year) can be managed medically without need for referral to cardiac catheterization (strength of evidence = B).

Recommendation: Patients with a high-risk exercise test result (predicted average annual cardiac mortality ≥4%/year) should be referred for prompt cardiac catheterization (strength of evidence = B).

Recommendation: Patients with intermediate-risk exercise test results (predicted average annual cardiac mortality 2 to 3%/year) should be referred for additional testing, either cardiac catheterization or an (alternative) exercise imaging study (strength of evidence = C).

Table 16.   Noninvasive studies in patients with unstable angina reporting at least 10 cardiac events (cardiac death or myocardial infarction) during followup

	Study	Inclusion criteria	Low risk	High risk
A	Moss, Goldstein, Hall et al, 1993	30% Unstable angina; 26% Non-Q-wave MI	893	23
B	Swahn, Areskog, Berglund et al, 1987	All unstable angina	247	145
C	Severi, Orsini, Marraccini et al, 1988	All unstable angina	199	175
D	Madsen, Thomsen, Mellerngaard et al, 1988	All unstable angina	118	98
E	Nyman, Larsson, Areskog et al, 1992	All unstable angina	366	374
F	Krone, Dwyer, Greenberg et al, 1989	All non-Q-wave MI	85	7
A	Moss, Goldstein, Hall et al, 1993	30% Unstable angina; 26% Non-Q-wave MI	876	20
D	Madsen, Thomsen, Mellerngaard et al, 1988	All unstable angina	129	29
G	Gibson, Beller, Gheorghiade et al, 1986	Non-Q-wave MI; 64% MI	133	108
H	Younis, Byers, Shaw et al, 1989	58% Unstable angina, 42% MI	14	54

Recommendation: A stress test result of intermediate risk combined with evidence of LV dysfunction should prompt referral to cardiac catheterization (strength of evidence = C).

Noninvasive tests are most useful in patient management decisions when risk can be stated in terms of events over time. A large population of patients must be studied to derive and test equations needed to accurately predict risk for individ-

The major question in this section is who should be evaluated by noninvasive testing. The guideline takes the approach of describing who is not suitable for noninvasive testing and assumes that all others are. This approach is somewhat obtuse and rarely followed in practice. The guideline states that those with a very low likelihood of coronary disease and at low risk of an event would not be subjected to noninvasive testing, because even if the test was positive, the index of suspicion would be so low that they would not undergo further evaluation with coronary angiography. In today's litigious atmosphere this advice would not be followed. Almost all such patients would at least have an ECG exercise test and anyone with a positive stress test would have an imaging stress test or be given consideration for catheterization. The few patients with positive tests who do not undergo cardiac catheterization would still be given intensive risk-factor counseling, as if they had CAD. Thus, the real answer to the question, with very few exceptions, is that everyone who does not have cardiac catheterization should get a noninvasive test.

The next issue is what type of noninvasive test to perform. There are 2 criteria here—one is the type of stress, and the second is the type of ischemia detection system. Exercise is almost always the best stress to employ, unless the patient cannot exercise or it is believed that the patient cannot perform well on exercise testing. In such situations, pharmacologic stress testing should be used. Some argue that an imaging stress test always gives better diagnostic or prognostic information than the standard ECG stress test. Although this may be true, it is a more expensive approach and if false-positive results are obtained, then the patient almost always has to go to cardiac catheterization, because there is no further escalation of noninvasive testing. Thus, ECG exercise stress testing should be done first in anyone who can exercise and has a normal resting ECG. If the patient exercises well and has a negative ECG response, then even if he or she has coronary artery disease the risk of an event is low and the prognosis is good. Those with a positive ECG response, chest pain, or other signs of ischemia, such as hypotension, would then be referred for cardiac catheterization if appropriate. Those in whom there are some minor ECG changes during exercise, but no other signs of myocardial ischemia, in whom a false-positive response is suspected, could then be exercised with myocardial imaging.

If a patient is going to have a myocardial imaging test performed, which imaging modality should be chosen? The guideline states that this depends on local expertise and the technologies available. I would add to this the cost of each of the imaging modalities at the institution in question and the quality of the service obtained from the imaging laboratory. When evaluating

(Continued)

(Continued from previous page)

unstable angina patients, long delays to obtain imaging stress tests are not acceptable. Beyond these considerations it is difficult to choose between echocardiography and myocardial nuclear perfusion imaging testing modalities. Most agree that radionuclide angiography is no longer considered the best imaging technique for evaluating patients with suspected or overt coronary disease. Better diagnostic sensitivities and specificities are obtained with other imaging techniques and the prognostic information available from radionuclide angiography can be obtained by other methods. The most popular imaging test is nuclear perfusion imaging, although some believe that in women or patients with LBBB, echocardiography provides fewer false-positive examinations. This conclusion has not been rigorously tested and the considerations above would probably take precedence over others.

When pharmacologic stress testing is to be employed, the type of imaging selected determines the pharmacologic agent to be used. Echocardiography should only be used with dobutamine or other pressor-type stressors. Although there has been some success with the vasodilator drugs dipyridamole and adenosine with echocardiographic imaging, in general the results are not as good as with dobutamine or other catecholamine-type stimulants. On the other hand, nuclear perfusion imaging is best done with vasodilators, such as dipyridamole or adenosine. The choice between dipyridamole and adenosine is still being evaluated. Dipyridamole causes fewer side effects, but these effects last longer and often require an aminophylline infusion to reverse them; adenosine produces more side effects, but these effects are of much shorter duration and do not require antidotes.

ual patients. No noninvasive study has been reported in a sufficient number of patients after stabilization of unstable angina to develop and test the accuracy of a multivariable equation to report test results in terms of absolute risk. Therefore, data borrowed from studies of patients with stable angina must be used if risk is to be reported as events/time. Although the pathologic process evoking ischemia may be different in the two subgroups, it is likely that use of prognostic nomograms derived on groups of patients with stable angina would also be predictive of risk in patients with recent unstable angina after stabilization. Using this untested assumption, the much larger literature derived from populations that include patients with both stable and unstable angina provides equations for risk stratification which convert physiologic changes observed during noninvasive testing into statements of risk expressed as events over time.

An exercise treadmill is the most commonly used stress test and has the largest reported experience for use in patients with unstable angina. A nomogram useful

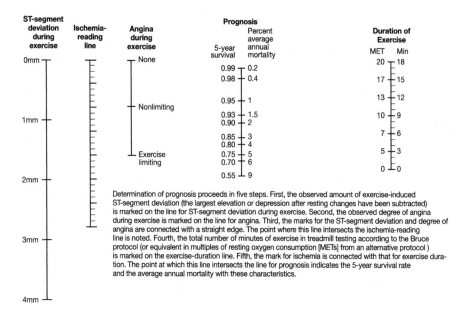

Determination of prognosis proceeds in five steps. First, the observed amount of exercise-induced ST-segment deviation (the largest elevation or depression after resting changes have been subtracted) is marked on the line for ST-segment deviation during exercise. Second, the observed degree of angina during exercise is marked on the line for angina. Third, the marks for the ST-segment deviation and degree of angina are connected with a straight edge. The point where this line intersects the ischemia-reading line is noted. Fourth, the total number of minutes of exercise in treadmill testing according to the Bruce protocol (or equivalent in multiples of resting oxygen consumption [METs] from an alternative protocol) is marked on the exercise-duration line. Fifth, the mark for ischemia is connected with that for exercise duration. The point at which this line intersects the line for prognosis indicates the 5-year survival rate and the average annual mortality with these characteristics.

Figure 11.   Nomogram of the prognostic relations embodied in the treadmill score.

to convert results from this test into a statement of mortality has been derived on a large sample of patients with CAD (Figure 11). Even though use of this nomogram to quantitate risk from results of treadmill examinations may understate risk in patients with unstable angina, this approach provides more clinically useful information than a simple normal/abnormal reading (Mark, Shaw, Harrell et al., 1991).

Patient Counseling

Results of a noninvasive test should be reported to the patient, his or her family, and advocate in language they can understand, and the test results should be used by the patient and the doctor to determine the advisability of cardiac catheterization and the need for adjustments in the patient's medical regimen.

Medical Record

The medical record should include:

■ Indications for test.

■ Type of test performed.

■ Summary of test results including ECG changes, symptoms, hemodynamic changes, reason for termination (exercise tests).

■ Test complications.

■ Summary of post-test prognosis (low-, intermediate-, high-risk or probability of adverse-event calculation).

7

Guideline: Cardiac Catheterization and Myocardial Revascularization

Commentary by Craig Timm, M.D.

Introduction

Cardiac catheterization does not directly benefit patient outcome, and its value as a diagnostic test derives from the detailed structural and functional information it provides that allows the clinician to assess prognosis accurately and to select the most appropriate long-term management strategy. Therefore, indications to use this procedure are interwoven with indications for possible therapeutic plans such as PTCA or CABG.

Patients come to cardiac catheterization for several indications that may develop at any time during the initial hospitalization for unstable angina. Cardiac catheterization is usually indicated in patients who fail to stabilize with medical therapy or have break-through symptoms despite adequate medical therapy, and in high-risk patients categorized by other clinical findings or noninvasive testing. Other possible indications for catheterization include significant CHF, malignant ventricular arrhythmias, significant LV dysfunction or large perfusion defect by noninvasive study, or physical examination, or echocardiographic evidence of significant MR, aortic stenosis, or hypertrophic cardiomyopathy. Finally, patients in an intermediate- or high-risk category with previous PTCA or CABG should generally be considered for cardiac catheterization, unless prior catheterization data indicate that no further revascularization is likely to be technically possible (Figure 12).

In all cases, the general indications for catheterization and revascularization are tempered by individual patient characteristics and preferences. In the very frail elderly and in those with serious comorbid conditions, patient and physician judgments about risks and benefits are particularly important.

Objectives of Care

The purpose of cardiac catheterization is to provide detailed data about the size and distribution of coronary vessels, the location and extent of atherosclerotic disease in the coronary arteries, the extent of focal and global LV dysfunction, and the presence and severity of coexisting cardiac disorders (such as valvular or congenital lesions).

Revascularization refers to a set of procedures (both percutaneous and surgical) that have as their principal goal restoration, to the extent possible, of normal arterial blood flow to the myocardium. Although general guidelines can be offered, the decision to refer a patient for a revascularization procedure and the selection of the appropriate procedure both require the exercise of clinical judgment and thorough counseling with the patient and his or her family regarding the expected risks and benefits.

Approach to Care Objectives

Cardiac Catheterization

This guideline proposes two alternative definitive treatment strategies termed "early invasive" and "early conservative." Randomized trial data did not support the inherent superiority of either strategy based on medical outcomes (TIMI IIIB, 1994). The decision about which strategy to pursue for a given patient should be based on the patient's estimated risk (Chapter 1), available facilities, and patient preference. These strategies are defined below.

Recommendation: In the early invasive strategy, cardiac catheterization is performed routinely in all hospitalized patients without contraindications, usually within 48 hours of presentation (strength of evidence = A).

Recommendation: In the early conservative strategy, cardiac catheterization is performed routinely in patients admitted to the hospital with unstable angina who are candidates for a revascularization procedure and have one or more of the following high-risk indicators: prior revascularization (PTCA or CABG); associated CHF or depressed LV function (EF <0.50) by noninvasive study; malignant ventricular arrhythmia; persistent or recurrent pain/ischemia; and/or a functional study indicating high risk (strength of evidence = A).

Recommendation: Diagnostic catheterization should not be performed on patients with extensive comorbidity in whom the likely benefits of revascularization in terms of length and quality of life would not outweigh the risks (strength of evidence = B).

The proper role and timing of cardiac catheterization in unstable angina remains controversial. Diagnostic catheterization benefits patients primarily by enhancing the accuracy of prognostic stratification which can be used to adjust med-

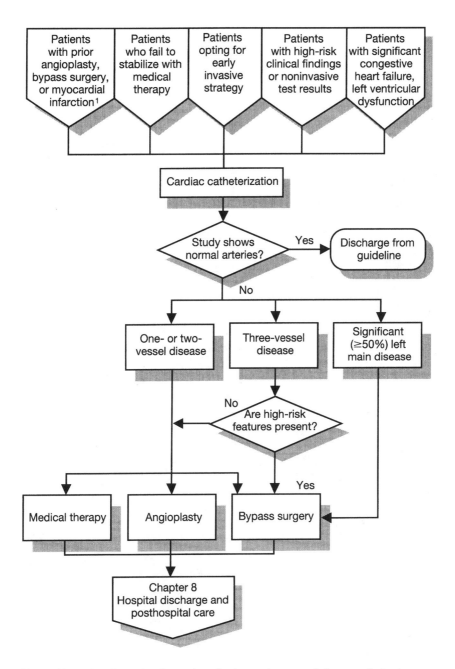

Figure 12. Patient flow: Cardiac catheterization and myocardial revascularization
[1]Those patients who are candidates for revascularization.

Numerous early studies on patients with acute MI included protocol-driven catheterization followed by coronary angioplasty if anatomy was suitable. These studies of mandated interventions showed no benefit and in some cases harm from the invasive procedures. As a result routine cardiac catheterization became somewhat discredited along with revascularization. Although not tested as a strategy in those early studies, the policy of cardiac catheterization alone followed by another decision point concerning revascularization has gained increased acceptance in acute MI patients. This acceptance has been aided by the low risk of a diagnostic catheterization procedure along with the added value of the procedure itself to both the patient (in terms of reassurance, necessity of life style modification, etc.) and the physician (choice of best therapy, information to help advise patient, etc.) This policy may be advisable in select patients with unstable angina, as well. In fact, on page 118 of this guideline document, it states that "after patients are hemodynamically stable on an appropriate initial medical regimen, consideration should be given to early invasive management (strength of evidence = A)." The guideline goes on to state that this point is usually within 48 hours for high-risk unstable angina patients, with consideration given to the later performance of bypass surgery or angioplasty.

At this point it is worth emphasizing the importance of including the patient and his or her family at all stages of the decisionmaking process. This is important because of the risk associated with invasive procedures, and because informed consent always requires patient understanding and input. Equally important is the goal of having the patient participate in the decision about diagnostic and therapeutic procedures when the indications are debatable due to lack of sufficient data from available clinical studies. In such cases the physician should aim to educate the patient about risks and benefits of the alternatives without interjecting his or her own biases. Reasonable and informed patients may make very different choices based on their own experiences and values. There is concern that the physician may use this opportunity to manipulate certain patients towards choosing an invasive approach, since patient preference is one of the indications for cardiac catheterization (see Figure 12). Many adequately informed patients do not have strong preferences and rely on the physician to make such decisions. In such cases it is important for the physician to make reasonable decisions based on evidence and experience.

Natural history studies have produced strong evidence that high-risk patients (Table 8) and some intermediate-risk patients are likely to develop adverse cardiac outcomes without intervention. Based on this evidence there is general agreement that such patients should undergo early catheterization and consideration of revascularization (Table 17). These patients are not generally included in therapeutic trials such as TIMI IIIB (1994).

ical therapy as well as to plan specific revascularization therapy. The population of patients with unstable angina admitted to the hospital includes a subgroup that should routinely receive catheterization and another subgroup for whom invasive study is optional and can be deferred pending further clinical developments. The group that should routinely receive catheterization consists of all high-risk patients (see Table 9) and intermediate-risk patients with a prior PTCA or CABG, patients with CHF or depressed resting LV function (i.e., EF <0.50) by noninvasive study, and patients recognized to be high risk by noninvasive exercise or pharmacologic stress testing. Decisions about catheterization in the low- or moderate-risk patients who also have a low-risk functional test can be individualized based on the practice setting (i.e., availability of invasive diagnostic and therapeutic procedures) and the patient's preferences.

The principal data upon which these recommendations are based are the TIMI IIIB (1994) results. This study randomized 1,473 patients with unstable angina requiring hospital admission to early (18 to 48 hours) invasive or early conservative strategies. At 42 days, 15.5 percent of the early invasive patients had died, had a nonfatal MI, or had a positive 6-week exercise test versus 17.7 percent of the early conservative patients (p = 0.26). Ninety-seven percent of the invasive group underwent diagnostic catheterization (as assigned) compared with 64 percent of the conservative group (p <0.001). Revascularization by 42 days had been performed in 61 percent of the invasive group and 49 percent of the conservative group (p

Table 17. Indications for cardiac catheterization in unstable angina

Prior MI or revascularization
Continued symptoms despite therapy
High- or intermediate-risk stress tests
Heart failure or LV dysfunction
Malignant arrhythmias
Rest angina <48 hours
Reversible ECG changes

The TIMI IIIB data have now been published including 42 day (TIMI IIIB, 1994) and 1 year (Anderson, Cannon, Stone et al., 1995) followup. Management of patients through the 42-day endpoint was according to protocol. Subsequently patient care was at the discretion of the physician. By protocol virtually all patients in the invasive arm had catheterization (97% at 42 days and 99% at 1 year) and, not surprisingly, a large portion subsequently underwent revascularization (61% at 42 days and 64% at 1 year). The crossover rate from conservative to invasive strategy was surprisingly high. At 42 days 64 percent of the conservative group had already had catheterization and 49 percent revascularization. These numbers increased to 73 percent and 58 percent at 1 year. The lack of protocol-driven care after 42 days has been cited as a possible weakness of the study, leading to a higher incidence of subsequent catheterization and revascularization because of a potential invasive bias by the patient's physician. However, the data do not support this as a major source of crossovers since at 6 weeks in the conservative arm 88 percent of catheterizations and 84 percent of revascularization procedures that would ultimately occur had already taken place.

<0.001). In addition, conservatively treated patients had a significantly higher use of antianginal medications and more hospital readmissions by the 6-week followup.

Although data are not available to permit a formal cost-effectiveness analysis of these alternate strategies, any savings realized initially in the group not receiving cardiac catheterization appear to be largely offset by the need for longer hospitalization initially and for subsequent care. Unless continued followup of these patients shows late survival benefit for patients treated by the early invasive strategy, the aggressiveness of early use of cardiac catheterization and revascularization procedures would appear to be best determined by the preferences of the individual patient with unstable angina.

At this time full data assessing cost of the TIMI IIIB (1994) strategies have still not been published. The early invasive arm is assumed to have somewhat higher initial costs based on more procedures. This may be offset somewhat at 6 weeks by excess hospitalization days for readmission and by excess noninvasive testing in the conservative arm. And though data are not available, it appears that this gap will be even further narrowed at 1 year due to crossover to catheterization and revascularization procedures in the conservative group. Thus, it is unlikely that there will be major cost differences between the two strategies.

> Because patients with prior revascularization are at higher risk for ischemia-related problems they are generally excluded from studies such as TIMI IIIB (1994). Cardiac catheterization is considered the fastest and most cost effective way to obtain diagnosis in this subset of unstable angina patients.

Patients who present with intermediate- or high-risk unstable angina and a history of a prior PTCA within the past year have a high incidence of restenosis which often can be effectively treated by repeat angioplasty. Noninvasive testing is not sufficiently accurate to detect restenosis in these patients, and coronary angiography without preceding functional testing is generally indicated. Patients with prior CABG surgery and intermediate- or high-risk unstable angina represent a second group for whom a strategy of early coronary angiography is generally indicated. In patients with recent bypass, early graft stenosis frequently can be treated with angioplasty. The complex interplay between progression of native coronary disease, development of graft atherosclerosis with ulceration and embolization, and the potential for noncardiac chest pain all argue for a greater need to visualize coronary arteries by catheterization in patients with prior bypass surgery than in patients with similar presenting symptoms but no prior procedure.

Patients with CAD and known or suspected poor LV function, such as patients with known prior Q-wave MIs or those who have had prior measurements of LV function or who present with CHF, have sufficient probability of benefit from revascularization procedures to merit direct coronary angiography without preceding functional testing.

Confirmation of normalcy in patients presenting frequently with symptoms of unstable angina and no objective evidence of ischemia represents another valid indication for cardiac catheterization. Identification and management of this patient group is described more fully in Chapter 3.

> As mentioned in earlier comments, patient participation in decisionmaking is imperative. This applies to cardiac catheterization as well as revascularization procedures. Some patients are easily reassured by a normal noninvasive test while others may continue to have episodes of chest pain prompting further outpatient/ED visits and hospitalizations. In such cases catheterization may be valuable to reassure the patient as well as direct future evaluation.

In unstable angina, results of catheterization typically show the following profile: (1) normal coronary arteries or insignificant CAD in 10 to 20 percent; (2) significant (i.e., >50%) left main disease in 5 to 10 percent; (3) three-vessel disease in 20 to 25 percent; (4) two-vessel disease in 25 to 30 percent; and (5) single-vessel disease in 30 to 35 percent. In the TIMI-IIIB (1994) early invasive strategy, no significant CAD >60 percent obstruction was found in 19 percent of patients, one-vessel disease in 38 percent, two-vessel disease in 29 percent, three-vessel disease in 15 percent, and left main disease (>50 percent obstruction) in 4 percent. Lesions are often eccentric with irregular borders in patients with unstable angina, and irregular lesion morphology has correlated with an increased risk of ischemia, MI, and cardiac death (Bugiardini, Pozzati, Borghi et al., 1991).

Discovery that a patient does not have significant obstructive CAD can help avert improper labeling and prompt a search for the true cause of symptoms. High-risk patients with two-vessel disease including patients with severe proximal LAD involvement, and those with severe three-vessel or left main disease should be considered for CABG. Many other patients will have less severe lesions that do not put them at high risk of cardiac death but can have a substantial negative impact on their quality of life. As compared with high-risk patients, low-risk patients will receive negligible or very modestly increased chances of long-term survival with CABG. Therefore, quality of life and patient preferences will be given more weight than strict clinical outcomes in selecting a treatment strategy. Low-risk patients whose symptoms do not respond well to maximal medical therapy and who experience a significant negative impact on their quality of life and functional status may be considered for revascularization. Patients in this group who are unwilling to accept the increased short-term procedural risks to gain long-term benefits or who are quite satisfied with their existing capabilities should be managed medically at first and followed carefully as outpatients. Other patients willing to accept the risks of revascularization and wishing to improve their functional status or to decrease symptoms may be considered appropriate candidates to undergo early elective revascularization.

It is not possible presently to define an arbitrary extent of comorbidity that would in every case make referral for cardiac catheterization and further invasive procedures inappropriate. As a general principle, the potential benefits of catheterization and revascularization must be carefully weighed against the risks which may be significantly greater in patients with significant comorbidity. This decision is further complicated because even when CABG surgery is not an option, high-risk patients may benefit from a palliative PTCA or other interventional procedure.

The case of the high-risk patient with significant comorbidities calls for especially thoughtful discussion between the health care practitioner, patient, and family. The decision for or against revascularization should be made on a case-by-case basis, and all parties should be in mutual agreement. Patients and families should

A recent study (Morrison, Sacks et al., 1995) reported on the use of PT-CA in a group of veterans with unstable angina who were considered high risk for CABG due to the presence of one or more of the following: prior CABG, age >70, EF <35%, MI within 7 days, use of IV NTC within 48 hours, or need for IABP. These 6 factors were selected because of excess CABG mortality in prior Veterans Administration studies. Two hundred seven patients with unstable angina met these criteria. Success rate and details of angioplasty procedures are not given. Mortality was 5 percent, and 90 percent of all patients were free of angina at discharge. Two year mortality was 18 percent, similar to the 21 percent 2 year CABG mortality in high-risk patients. It may be difficult to extrapolate these results to other potential high-risk situations. However, these data support the utility of PTCA in the Veterans Administration high-risk patients and the value of proceeding to cardiac catheterization with the hope of finding lesions suitable for PTCA.

understand that the presence of significant comorbidities can alter the revascularization risk-to-benefit ratio and negatively influence patient outcomes.

Examples of extensive comorbidity within the spirit of this recommendation include:

- Advanced or metastatic malignancy with a projected life expectancy ≤1 year.
- Intracranial pathology contraindicating the use of systemic anticoagulation.
- End-stage hepatic cirrhosis with symptomatic portal hypertension (e.g., encephalopathy, visceral bleeding).

This list is not meant to be all-inclusive, and clinical judgment must be exercised in identifying other types of extensive comorbidity.

More difficult decisions involve patients with significant comorbidity but not as significant as described above. Examples of this group of patients include those with:

- Moderate or severe renal insufficiency.
- Hepatic cirrhosis with functional hepatic insufficiency.

Precatheterization consultation with an interventional cardiologist and a cardiac surgeon is advised to define the technical options open to the patient and the likely risks and benefits of each.

The nature of the facility performing the catheterization also can be an important consideration in this evaluation. Specifically, the availability of interventional cardiologists experienced in high-risk and palliative PTCA should be considered, as should the availability of an experienced cardiac surgeon able and willing to take on complex, high-risk cases.

Revascularization

Recommendation: Consideration should be given to the possibility of non-coronary symptom etiologies in patients found at catheterization to have normal coronary arteries or insignificant lesions (<70% stenosis) (strength of evidence = C).

Recommendation: Patients found at catheterization to have significant left main disease (≥50%) or significant (≥70%) three-vessel disease with depressed LV function (EF <0.50) should be referred promptly for CABG surgery (strength of evidence = A).

Recommendation: Patients with two-vessel disease with proximal severe subtotal stenosis (≥95%) of the LAD and depressed LV function should be referred promptly for revascularization (strength of evidence = B for CABG; strength of evidence = C for PTCA).

Recommendation: Patients with significant CAD should be considered for prompt revascularization (PTCA or CABG) if they have any of the following: failure to stabilize with medical treatment; recurrent angina/ischemia at rest or with low-level activities; and/or ischemia accompanied by CHF symptoms, an S_3 gallop, new or worsening MR, or definite ECG changes (strength of evidence = B).

Recommendation: For patients with significant CAD not included in the above recommendations, two strategies are possible: early invasive and early conservative. In the early invasive strategy, CABG or PTCA is performed. In the early conservative strategy, revascularization is performed only on those patients meeting criteria for failure of initial therapy necessitating cardiac catheterization. Medical therapy without revascularization is continued for patients without criteria for failure of therapy (strength of evidence = A).

Revascularization is used to improve prognosis, relieve symptoms, and improve functional capacity in patients with obstructive CAD. In general, the indications for revascularization in the unstable angina patient who has been stabilized are the same as for stable angina, but the impetus for some form of revascularization is stronger than in stable angina. Moreover, long-term survival rates after CABG are similar for unstable angina patients who present with rest angina, in-

In patients for whom the indications for revascularization are less clear, the angiographic morphology of coronary stenoses may be an additional factor to consider. Natural history studies have shown that patients whose lesions have a complex morphology (irregular borders, overhanging edges, or intra-coronary thrombus) are at higher risk for subsequent cardiac complications than those whose lesions have smooth borders. Adverse cardiac in-hospital endpoints were measured and included MI, sudden death, and emergency revascularization. Fifty-five percent of patients with complex morphology had an adverse endpoint compared to only 6 percent of patients with smooth stenoses.

The Thrombolysis and Angioplasty in Unstable Angina (TAUSA) trial reported on the outcome of angioplasty of complex lesions in unstable angina patients (Mehran, Ambrose, et al., 1995). Complex morphology was defined as above. Compared to smooth lesions, complex lesions had a higher abrupt closure rate (10.6% vs. 3.3%, $p < 0.003$) and a higher emergency bypass surgery rate (5.2% vs. 0.9%, $p < 0.02$). This indicates a higher risk for complex lesion morphology whether the patient is revascularized or not. This is expected given the active, thrombogenic milieu associated with complex lesions. Nonetheless, the balance appears to be in favor of intervention. While a recommendation cannot be made for intervention based on morphology alone, it may be a useful additional factor to consider when the indications are unclear.

creasing angina, new onset angina, or post-MI angina (Rahimtoola, Nunley, Grunkemeier et al., 1983).

CABG and PTCA are the two revascularization strategies available, and implicit in this guideline is the understanding that the initial treatment selection will be modified or supplemented when necessitated by changes in the patient's condition. Thus, subsequent referrals of a PTCA patient to CABG surgery or of a CABG surgery patient to PTCA (i.e., therapeutic crossovers) are integral parts of the initial treatment strategy. However, excessive crossover rates suggest inappropriate treatment selection, inadequate technical results, or both. Furthermore, although the percutaneous intervention strategy is referred to in this guideline as "PTCA," it should be recognized that this term refers to a family of techniques including standard balloon angioplasty, perfusion balloon (prolonged dilatation) angioplasty, atherectomy, laser angioplasty, and intra-coronary stenting. Thus, once the decision has been made to attempt percutaneous coronary revascularization, a further decision is required about the optimal mode(s) of such intervention.

The TIMI-IIIB (1994) results comparing early invasive versus early conservative catheterization and revascularization have been described in the cardiac catheterization section of this chapter. Two randomized trials compared medical and surgical therapy in unstable angina. The National Cooperative Study Group randomized 288 patients between 1972 and 1976 at nine academic centers (Russell, Moraski, Kouchoukos, 1978). The Veterans Administration Cooperative Study randomized 468 patients between 1976 and 1982 at 12 VA hospitals (Luchi, Scott, and Deupree, 1987; Parisi, Khuri, Deupree et al., 1989; Scott, Luchi, and Deupree, 1988; Sharma, Deupree, Khuri et al., 1991). Both studies included patients with progressive or rest angina accompanied by ST- and T-wave changes. Patients over age 70 or with a recent MI were excluded. The VA study included only men.

In the National Cooperative Study, hospital mortality was 3 percent for medicine and 5 percent for CABG surgery (p = NS). Followup to 30 months failed to show any differences in survival between the therapies. In the VA study, survival to 2 years was the same for medicine and CABG surgery overall and in subgroups defined by number of diseased vessels. A post-hoc analysis of patients with depressed LV function, however, showed a significant survival advantage with CABG surgery. All randomized trials of CABG surgery versus medicine (including those in stable angina) have found improved symptom relief and functional capacity with CABG surgery. Long-term followup in these trials has suggested that by 10 years there is a significant attenuation of both symptom relief and survival benefits from CABG surgery. However, these randomized trials reflect an earlier technical era for both CABG surgery and medicine. Improvements in anesthesia and surgical techniques, including internal mammary artery grafting to the LAD artery and improved intra-operative myocardial protection with cold potassium cardioplegia, are not reflected in these trials. Also, the routine use of heparin and ASA in the acute phase and the range of therapeutic agents available represent significant differences in current practice from the era in which these trials were performed.

Three published and two unpublished randomized trials of PTCA have now been reported, but only one of these, the Randomized Intervention Treatment of

---

The VA study indicated above (Scott, Lurchi, Deupress, 1988) has now been published as a full paper (Scott et al., 1994) and confirms that the surgical advantage in patients with reduced LV ejection fraction is maintained to 8 years of followup, but changes at 10 years. Also, a recent report from the Coronary Artery Surgery Study (Cameron, Davis, Green, and Schaff, 1996) detailed the benefits of internal mammary grafts compared to vein grafting in that study population. The presence of a mammary graft was independently associated with an improved and increasing survival benefit over time. At 15 years the relative risk of death was 0.73 in patients with mammary grafts compared with vein grafts alone.

Angina (RITA), enrolled unstable angina patients. The VA Angioplasty Compared with Medicine (ACME) trial tested PTCA versus medicine in single-vessel disease and found improved functional status and quality of life at 6 months in the PTCA arm (Parisi, Folland, Hartigan et al., 1992). The RITA trial enrolled 1,011 patients in the United Kingdom with one-, two-, or three-vessel disease that had equal chance of revascularization success with either PTCA or CABG (RITA, 1993). Approximately 60 percent of the enrolled patients were reported to have angina at rest prior to randomization. An interim analysis at 2.5 years of followup has shown equivalent hard cardiac events (death, MI) and a much higher repeat revascularization rate in the PTCA arm. The German Angioplasty Bypass Surgery Investigation (GABI), which randomized 358 patients with multivessel CAD and ≥class II angina to CABG or multivessel PTCA, recently reported that at 6-month followup, the primary endpoint (angina rates) was similar, and there was no significant difference in the rates of hard cardiac events (death, MI) between the CABG and PTCA groups. Initial results have recently been presented for the Coronary Artery Bypass Revascularization Investigation (CABRI) trial involving 1,054 multivessel CAD patients randomized to PTCA or CABG. The Emory Angioplasty vs. Surgery Trial (EAST) also reported, but has not published, outcomes in 392 patients with multivessel disease, including a majority of patients with unstable angina, randomized between PTCA and CABG. The reported results of these two unpublished trials do not differ substantially from the reported results of the RITA trial.

One large registry compared 5-year survival with medicine, PTCA, and CABG in 9,263 CAD patients with unstable angina (defined as symptoms requiring hospital admission for control and to rule out MI) treated between 1984 and 1990 (Mark, Nelson, Califf et al., 1994). In this nonrandomized comparison, extensive statistical adjustments were used to control for prognostically important baseline differences created by treatment selection. For patients with three-vessel disease or two-vessel disease with a proximal severe (≥95%) LAD artery stenosis; surgical survival at 5 years was significantly better than medicine, and a similar trend in favor of CABG was found in comparison with PTCA. In less severe two-vessel CAD, revascularization improved survival relative to medicine, and there was a trend for PTCA to provide better survival results (due to lower procedural mortality) than CABG. In one-vessel disease, all therapies were associated with high 5-year survival rates with very small differences among groups.

The available data can be used to formulate some general principles about the proper role of revascularization in acute IHD. The first general principle is the more extensive the CAD, the larger the benefit in survival realized from revascularization (Califf, Harrell, Lee et al., 1989). In the most severe forms of CAD (e.g., left main disease, three-vessel disease), CABG provides the best long-term survival results. In intermediate forms of CAD (e.g., two-vessel disease), revascularization provides improved survival relative to medicine, although the absolute survival benefit is smaller than in three-vessel disease. In general, the patient with

Results at 3 years for the EAST study (King, Lembo et al., 1994) and at 1 year for the GABI study (Hamm, Reimers et al., 1994) have been published since the development of this guideline. As noted there are no significant differences in the hard cardiovascular endpoints at the time of followup. The reports indicate that unstable angina patients were in fact randomized (62% of patients had Class IV angina in EAST and 14% of patients had unstable angina in GABI). Separate outcomes are not reported for these subsets of patients.

While cardiac outcomes are not apparently different in these studies it is important to note that many more patients were screened than enrolled. In EAST over 5,000 patients with multivessel disease who had not previously had PTCA or CABG were screened. Three hundred ninety-two patients were ultimately enrolled. Major sources of exclusion included left main disease, chronic total occlusions, and severely reduced LV function. These patients were presumably treated with CABG. In GABI a large number of patients was excluded for similar reasons. So even though PTCA and CABG have similar outcomes in these studies, the number of such patients to whom PTCA and CABG are equally viable options is smaller than it appears since many high-risk or technically unsuitable patients will preferably be offered CABG.

high-risk two-vessel disease (as defined by impaired LV function, older age, or co-existing vascular disease) will have improved survival with CABG surgery as compared with other patients who have two-vessel disease and similar anatomy. For other two-vessel disease patients, PTCA may provide modest survival benefits relative to medicine. In the least severe CAD patients (i.e., one-vessel disease), observational data have shown good survival associated with medical therapy, PTCA, and CABG. The primary treatment choice is usually between medicine and PTCA, with CABG reserved for those patients with large areas of myocardium at risk, those who fail medical therapy, or those who are technically unsuitable for PTCA.

The second general principle is that survival benefits of revascularization are magnified on the absolute scale by factors that increase overall medical risk, especially LV dysfunction and advanced age. In particular, multivessel CAD benefits from CABG are substantially larger on an absolute scale in patients with depressed LV function. These factors tend to increase the procedural risks of revascularization somewhat but offer proportionally greater long-term benefits than can be expected with medical treatment (Califf, Harrell, Lee et al., 1989; McCormick, Schick, McCabe et al., 1985).

These general principles in the revascularization guideline offer an excellent summary (Table 18). It is possible that future randomized studies will show PTCA to be equivalent to CABG in high-risk patients with multivessel disease and reduced LV function. However, based on current knowledge, CABG is best suited for these patients. Patients with intermediate risk may be offered either form of revascularization to obtain a survival advantage. Finally, lowest risk patients should be managed with the least risk initially (i.e., medical therapy), and then revascularization if unacceptable symptoms continue and the patient is willing to assume the risk. PTCA would of course be considered first given the lower initial morbidity.

As in many areas of medicine, the patient with the highest risk also stands to gain the most if treatment is successful. This is exemplified by the issues of multivessel disease and reduced LV function in an elderly patient. Unfortunately the price is paid up front in terms of procedural morbidity and mortality. It is thus essential for physician, patient, and family to agree that this risk is acceptable for the hope of improved longevity and quality of life.

Patient Counseling

Recommendation: The health care team should work with the patient, his or her family, and advocate to provide education about the expected risks and benefits of revascularization (CABG or PTCA) and to determine individual patient preferences and fears that can affect the selection of therapy. The health care team can use this opportunity to dispel incorrect assumptions or unreasonable fears held by the patient, family, or advocate. In addition, the patient should be informed of sensory experiences (e.g., what the patient will feel, hear, see, etc.) associated with the procedure, the usual expected recovery process, and any behaviors that the patient would be expected to perform to enhance recovery. The patient, family, and advocate should be given the opportunity to have their questions answered and to express their concerns (strength of evidence = B).

Table 18.   General indications for revascularization

Refractory angina plus severe coronary obstruction
Multivessel disease with reduced LV function
Aortic stenosis and CAD
Left main disease ($\geq$narrowing)
High-risk patients with appropriate coronary anatomy

The decision between angioplasty, bypass surgery, or medical treatment is a difficult one for many patients. Many patients fear death or disability from surgery more than from the progression of their disease. Other patients view bypass surgery as a panacea for their condition that will allow them to avoid difficult changes in their present lifestyle, even though a repeat procedure may be needed later. All care providers, especially physicians directly responsible for care during procedures, should provide a balanced and accurate summary of risks and benefits of all reasonable therapeutic options.

Patient expectations regarding the benefits of revascularization are quite variable. In one study, bypass patients were asked before their surgery about the benefits they expected to obtain (Gortner, Gilliss, Paul et al., 1989). Six months later, they were resurveyed to determine which benefits had been achieved. Women realized fewer expected benefits than men (62% vs. 90%, p <0.05). In addition, younger patients realized fewer expected benefits than older patients. Often the patients held unrealistic expectations. Assessment of expectations before a procedure may help a patient and physician make a more appropriate treatment decision.

Medical Record

The following information should be recorded in the medical record:

Reasons for cardiac catheterization.

- Cardiac catheterization findings summarized by number of major coronary arteries with 70 percent or greater stenosis, presence or absence of a 50 percent or greater left main stenosis, LV EF, and presence and severity of valvular disease.
- For patients undergoing interventional therapy, the primary reason for the procedure, indicated as enhanced survival, pain relief, both, or other.
- All complications, time of occurrence, and relationship to the procedure.
- Complications occurring during one procedure that led to another, different procedure (such as angioplasty failure leading to CABG surgery) including assessment of their severity at the beginning of the second procedure.
- Deaths classified as noncardiac or cardiac.
- Cardiac deaths classified as precipitated by arrhythmia, progressive ischemia, or progressive cardiac failure.

8

Guideline:
Hospital Discharge
and Postdischarge Care

Commentary by Michael H. Crawford, M.D.

Background

The natural history of unstable angina is typically characterized by either progression to nonfatal MI or death on the one hand, or resumption of the more quiescent clinical course of chronic stable angina on the other. The acute phase of unstable angina is usually over within 8 weeks. The need for continued hospitalization of the unstable angina patient is determined by whether the inpatient objectives of that hospital admission have been achieved.

Patients who have undergone successful revascularization will usually have the remainder of their hospitalization defined by the standard protocol for the given procedure (e.g., 1 to 2 days for PTCA, 5 to 7 days for CABG surgery). Patients electing medical treatment after a cardiac catheterization or functional study include both a low-risk group that can be rapidly discharged (e.g., 1 to 2 days after testing) and a high-risk group unsuitable for or unwilling to have coronary revascularization. These latter patients may require a prolonged hospitalization to ensure adequate (or as adequate as possible) symptom control and that risk of cardiac events in the next 4 to 6 weeks has fallen to an acceptably low level.

Management of all these patient groups prior to hospital discharge is described in the preceding chapters. Details and objectives of care from the time of hospital discharge until the final clinic visit for the unstable angina episode are described in this chapter (Figure 13).

Objectives of Care

The goal during the hospital discharge phase is to prepare the patient for normal activities to the extent possible. The goal of postdischarge outpatient care is to make adjustments in the discharge regimen that appear most appropriate after

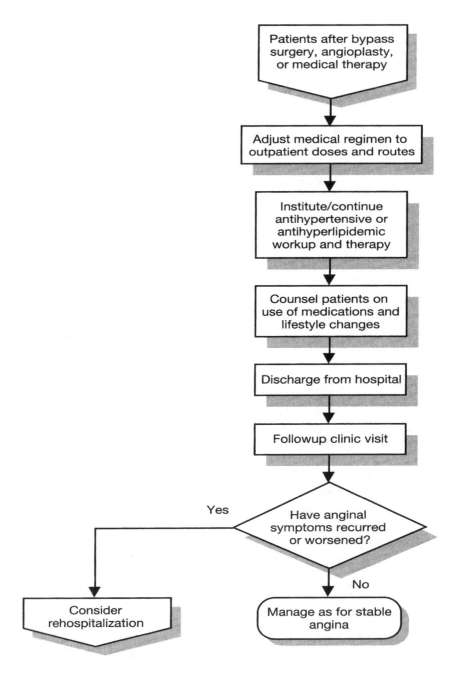

Figure 13. Patient flow: Hospital discharge and postdischarge care.

an initial period away from direct patient care. The long-term management of the unstable angina event ends as the patient re-enters the stable phase of CAD.

Approach to Care Objectives

Discharge Medical Regimen

Recommendation: Patients should continue on ASA, 80 mg to 324 mg per day, indefinitely after discharge (strength of evidence = B, evidence cited in Chapter 3).

Recommendation: In general, those classes of medications necessary to achieve adequate symptom control should be continued after discharge. Patients with successful revascularization without recurrent ischemia do not require postdischarge antianginal therapy. Patients with unsuccessful revascularization or with recurrent symptoms following revascularization should be continued on the regimen required in hospital to control their symptoms (strength of evidence = C).

Recommendation: All patients with signs and symptoms suggesting ongoing ischemia should be given sublingual NTG and instructed in its use (strength of evidence = C).

Recommendation: Antihypertensive and antihyperlipidemic workups and therapies started prior to admission or initiated in the hospital should be continued in the postdischarge phase (strength of evidence = C).

The use of and rationale for different medical agents have been described earlier in this guideline. In most cases, the inpatient medical regimen used in the non-intensive phase will be continued postdischarge. The need for continued medical therapy after discharge relates to potential prognostic benefits (primarily shown for ASA and beta blockers), control of symptoms (nitrates and calcium antagonists), and treatment of major risk factors, such as hypertension, hyperlipidemia, and diabetes mellitus. Thus, selection of a medical regimen will be individualized to the specific needs of each patient and the events that have occurred in hospital.

Discharge of a patient from the hospital often requires a team effort from the medical staff (physicians, nurses, dietitians, pharmacists, rehabilitation specialists, physical and occupational therapists). Use of instruction sheets can help to document and reinforce the instructions given but should not be used in lieu of in-person instruction.

Postdischarge Followup

Recommendation: The plan for followup medical care should be set, whenever possible, at the time of discharge (strength of evidence = C). In general, low-risk patients and patients with successful CABG or PTCA should be seen in an outpatient facility at 2 to 6 weeks, and higher risk patients should return in 1 to 2 weeks (strength of evidence = C).

Clinical information available at discharge has been shown by Cox analysis to predict death within 1 year in 515 survivors of hospitalization for non-Q-wave MI, including persistent ST-segment depression, CHF, advanced age, and ST-segment elevation (Schechtman, Capone, Kleiger et al., 1989). Patients with all high-risk markers present had a 14-fold increase in mortality compared with patients with all markers absent. Patients recognized to be at high risk for a cardiac event after discharge deserve earlier and more frequent followup than low-risk patients.

Recommendation: Patients with recurrent unstable angina should be managed as specified in an earlier chapter of this guideline corresponding to the clinical situation (strength of evidence = B, evidence cited in Chapter 6).

Recommendation: Patients who have stable or no anginal symptoms at this followup visit should be managed further for stable CAD (strength of evidence = C).

It is presently unclear whether patients who come through an episode of unstable angina without complications are at increased risk for future episodes of unstable angina, but their overall risk for death or MI is similar to that of other CAD patients with their characteristics who have not had unstable angina. The last element in the management of unstable angina, therefore, is a followup clinic visit at the point when the patient's disease activity has returned to the baseline level.

Patient Counseling

Use of Medications

Recommendation: The patient and his or her family members or advocate should be instructed in the purpose, dose, and major side effects of each medicine prescribed using language the patient can understand (strength of evidence = C).

Recommendation: Specific instructions for the proper use of sublingual NTG are especially important, since response of chest pain to this specific regimen is useful in assessing the nature of recurrent symptoms (strength of evidence = C).

Monitoring Symptoms

Recommendation: Because the hospital stay for unstable angina patients is often very short, it has been found that one way to increase patient compliance to the treatment regimen and risk-factor modification program is to provide telephone followup (strength of evidence = B).

Either formal or informal telephone followup can serve to reinforce in-hospital learning, provide reassurance, and answer the patient's questions. Beckie (1989) found that bypass patients in a telephone followup program telephoned their physicians less frequently and had fewer readmissions, lower anxiety, and higher CAD knowledge scores compared with the control group.

Where personnel and budget resources allow, the health care team may consider establishing such a followup system in which nurses telephone patients approximately once a week for the first 4 weeks after discharge. This structured program would gauge the progress of the patient's recovery, reinforce the CAD education taught in hospital, address patient questions and concerns, and monitor progress in meeting risk behavior modification goals.

Recommendation: Recurrent symptoms lasting more than 1 to 2 minutes should prompt the patient to stop his or her activities, sit down, and place an NTG tablet under the tongue. This may be repeated twice at 5-minute intervals for two additional tablets. If symptoms persist after three NTG tablets, the patient should promptly seek medical attention (strength of evidence = C).

Recommendation: If symptoms change in pattern (e.g., asymptomatic to symptomatic, more frequent or more severe symptoms), the patient should contact his or her primary care physician and discuss whether changes in the management plan are warranted. However, if the patient cannot reach a physician and chest pain persist for more than 20 minutes or despite three NTG tablets, he or she should seek transportation to the nearest hospital ED either by ambulance or the fastest available alternative (strength of evidence = C).

Activity Level and Lifestyle Changes

Recommendation: Specific instructions should be given on smoking cessation, daily exercise, and diet (strength of evidence = B). Where possible and appropriate, consideration should be given to referral to a smoking-cessation program or clinic and/or an outpatient cardiac rehabilitation program (strength of evidence = C).

The health care team should work with patients and their families to set specific goals for risk-factor reduction. In some cases, the family may be able and willing to support the patient further by also making changes in risk behaviors (e.g., cooking low-fat meals for the entire family, exercising together).

Particular attention should be paid to smoking cessation. Daly, Mulcahy, Graham, and colleagues (1983) measured the long-term effects of smoking on patients with unstable angina. For men under 60 years of age, those who continued to smoke had a risk of death from all causes 5.4 times that of men who stopped smoking ($p > 0.05$).

More specific recommendations on risk-factor modification and cardiac rehabilitation are beyond the scope of this guideline.

Since the publication of the unstable angina guideline, guidelines on cardiac rehabilitation have been published. They suggest that anybody with identified heart disease can benefit from cardiac rehabilitation. Unstable angina patients who have been stabilized and discharged certainly fall into this category. In addition to exercise rehabilitation, cardiac rehabilitation sessions should include education on risk-factor modification, from which many of these patients can benefit. Smoking cessation is extremely important, but the achievement of this goal is often difficult. Thus, there has been interest in the use of nicotine patches. The concern in patients who have been recently stabilized after a bout of unstable angina is that the potential heart rate and blood pressure effects of nicotine may actually aggravate or exaggerate their myocardial ischemia and angina. Getting the patient off cigarettes is a laudable long-term goal, but there may be some danger in the short term because of the pharmacologic effects of nicotine. Although this has not been studied in patients with heart disease, it is my opinion that nicotine patches should be avoided under these circumstances, unless the patient has been stabilized for a considerable period of time.

We usually advise our patients that they can resume sexual activity as soon as they feel up to it. Studies have shown that sex with a familiar partner, and doing other familiar activities is not particularly stressful and usually causes no problems in patients with ischemic heart disease. Sex with a new partner or engaging in activities to which the patient is unaccustomed is more likely to produce problems and should be avoided.

Recommendation: Health care providers should initiate a conversation with the patient to discuss the safety and timing of the resumption of sexual activity (e.g., 2 weeks for low-risk patients to 4 weeks for post-CABG surgery patients) (strength of evidence = C).

Very often patients will not ask their physicians or other health care providers about resuming sexual activity after their hospitalization. When appropriate, patients need to be reassured that sexual activity is still possible, and it is not likely to result in death or recurrent symptoms.

Recommendation: Beyond the instructions for daily exercise, patients require specific instruction on activities that are permissible and those that should be avoided (e.g., heavy lifting, climbing stairs, yard work, household activities). Specific mention should be made of resumption of driving and return to work (strength of evidence = C).

Medical Record

The patient's medical record from the time of hospital discharge should indicate the discharge medical regimen, the major instructions about postdischarge activities and rehabilitation, and the patient's understanding and plan for adherence to the recommendations. The medical record of the final outpatient visit after full resolution of the episode of unstable angina should summarize cardiac events, current symptoms, medication changes since hospital discharge or last outpatient visit, and document the plan for future care as a patient with stable CAD.

References

Note that bullet point (■) indicates material referenced by the editor—ed.

Aase O, Jonsbu J, Liestol K et al. Decision support by computer analysis of selected case history variables in the emergency room among patients with acute chest pain. Eur Heart J 1993 Apr;14:433–40.

Ahmed WH, Bittl JA, Braunwald E. Relation between clinical presentation and angiographic findings in unstable angina pectoris, and comparison with that in stable angina. Am J Cardiol 1993 Sep;72:544–50.

Amanullah A, Bevegard S, Lindvall K et al. Early exercise thallium-201 single photon emission computed tomography in unstable angina: a prospective study. Clin Physiol 1992 Nov;12:607–17.

Ambrose JA, Hjemdahl-Monsen CE, Borrico S et al. Angiographic demonstration of a common link between unstable angina pectoris and non-Q-wave acute myocardial infarction. Am J Cardiol 1988 Feb;61(4):244–7.

Ambrose JA, Torre SR, Sharma SK et al. Adjunctive thrombolytic therapy for angioplasty in ischemic rest angina: results of a double-blind randomized pilot study. J Am Coll Cardiol 1992 Nov;20:197–204.

■ Anderson HV, Cannon CP, Stone PH, et al. for the TIMI IIIB Investigators: One year results of the thrombolysis in myocardial infarction (TIMI) IIIB clinical trial. A randomized comparison of tissue-type plasminogen activator versus placebo and early invasive versus early conservative strategies in unstable angina and non-Q wave myocardial infarction. J Am Coll Cardiol 1995, 26:1643–50.

Antiplatelet Trialist's Collaboration. Collaborative overview of randomized trials of antiplatelet therapy. I. Prevention of death, myocardial infarction, and stroke by prolonged antiplatelet therapy in various categories of patients. Br Med J 1994; 308:81–106.

Arbustini E, Grasso M, Diegoli M et al. Coronary atherosclerotic plaques with and without thrombus in ischemic heart syndromes: a morphologic, immunohistochemical, and biochemical study. Am J Cardiol 1991 Sep;68(7):36B–50B.

Aroesty JM, Weintraub RM, Paulin S et al. Medically refractory unstable angina pectoris. II. Hemodynamic and angiographic effects of intraaortic balloon counterpulsation. Am J Cardiol 1979 May;43(5):883–8.

Balsano F, Rizzon P, Violi F et al. Antiplatelet treatment with ticlopidine in unstable angina. A controlled multicenter clinical trial. The Studio della Ticlopidina nell'Angina Instabile Group. Circulation 1990 Jul;82(1):17–26.

Bar FW, Verheugt FW, Col J et al. Thrombolysis in patients with unstable angina improves the angiographic but not the clinical outcome. Results of UNASEM, a multicenter, randomized, placebo-controlled, clinical trial with anistreplase. Circulation 1992 Jul;86:131–7.

Beckie T. A supportive-educative telephone program: impact on knowledge and anxiety after coronary artery bypass graft surgery. Heart Lung 1989 Jan;18(1):46–55.

Bosch X, Theroux P, Pelletier GB et al. Clinical and angiographic features and prognostic significance of early postinfarction angina with and without electrocardiographic signs of transient ischemia. Am J Med 1991 Nov;91(5):493–501.

Botker HE, Ravkilde J, Sogaard P et al. Gradation of unstable angina based on a sensitive immunoassay for serum creatine kinase MB. Br Heart J 1991 Feb;65:72–6.

Braunwald E. Unstable angina. A classification. Circulation 1989 Aug;80(2):410–4.

Brush JE Jr, Brand DA, Acampora D et al. Relation of peak creatine kinase levels during acute myocardial infarction to presence or absence of previous manifestations of myocardial ischemia (angina pectoris or healed myocardial infarction). Am J Cardiol 1988 Sep;62:534–7.

Bugiardini R, Pozzati A, Borghi A et al. Angiographic morphology in unstable angina and its relation to transient myocardial ischemia and hospital outcome. Am J Cardiol 1991 Mar;67:460–4.

Cairns JA, Gent M, Singer J et al. Aspirin, sulfinpyrazone, or both in unstable angina. Results of a Canadian multicenter trial. N Engl J Med 1985 Nov;313(22):1369–75.

Cairns JA, Singer J, Gent M et al. One year mortality outcomes of all coronary and intensive care unit patients with acute myocardial infarction unstable angina or other chest pain in Hamilton, Ontario, a city of 375,000 people. Can J Cardiol 1989 Jun;5:239–46.

Califf RM, Harrell FE, Lee KL et al. The evolution of medical and surgical therapy for coronary artery disease: A 15-year perspective. JAMA 1989 Apr;261(14):2077–86.

Califf RM, Mark DB, Harrell FE et al. Importance of clinical measures of ischemia in the prognosis of patients with documented coronary artery disease. J Am Coll Cardiol 1988 Jan;11(1):20–6.

■ Calvin JE, et al. Risk stratification in unstable angina. Prospective validation of the Braunwald classification. JAMA 1995 273:136–41.

■ Cameron A, Davis KB, Green G, and Schaff HV: Coronary bypass surgery with internal thoracic artery grafts—effects on survival over a 15 year period. N Engl J Med 1996 334:216–219.

Campeau L. Grading of angina pectoris [letter]. Circulation 1976 Sep;54(3):522–3.

CASS Group. Coronary artery surgery study (CASS), National Heart, Lung, and Blood Institute. Killip T, Fisher LD, Mock MB, eds. Circulation 1981;63(suppl 1):1–81.

Chaitman BR, Bourassa MG, Davis K et al. Angiographic prevalence of high-risk coronary artery disease in patient subgroups (CASS). Circulation 1981;64:360–7.

Charbonnier B, Bernadet P, Schiele F et al. Intravenous thrombolysis by recombinant plasminogen activator (rt-PA) in unstable angina. A randomized multicenter study versus placebo. Arch Mal Coeur Vaiss 1992 Oct;85:1471–7.

Cohen M, Hawkins L, Greenberg S et al. Usefulness of ST-segment changes in greater than or equal to 2 leads on the emergency room electrocardiogram in either unstable angina pectoris or non-Q-wave myocardial infarction in predicting outcome. Am J Cardiol 1991 Jun;67:1368–73.

Daly LE, Mulcahy R, Graham IM et al. Long term effect on mortality of stopping smoking after unstable angina and myocardial infarction. Br Med J 1983 July;287:324–6.

Davies MJ, Thomas A. Thrombosis and acute coronary-artery lesions in sudden cardiac ischemic death. N Engl J Med 1984 May;310(18):1137–40.

Dellborg M, Gustafsson G, Swedberg K. Buccal versus intravenous nitroglycerin in unstable angina pectoris. Eur J Clin Pharmacol 1991;41(1):5–9.

DePace NL, Herling IM, Kotler MN et al. Intravenous nitroglycerin for rest angina. Potential pathophysiologic mechanisms of action. Arch Intern Med 1982 Oct;142(10):1806–9.

De Servi S, Ghio S, Ragni T et al. Clinical, angiographic, and prognostic findings in unstable angina. G Ital Cardiol 1985;15(2):661–5.

■ de Winter RJ, et al. Value of myoglobin, tropinin T, and CK-MBmass in ruling out an acute myocardial infarction in the emergency room. Circulation 1995 92:3401–7.

Distante A, Maseri A, Severi S et al. Management of vasospastic angina at rest with continuous infusion of isosorbide dinitrate. A double crossover study in a coronary care unit. Am J Cardiol 1979 Sep;44(3):533–9.

Falk E. Morphologic features of unstable atherothrombotic plaques underlying acute coronary syndromes. Am J Cardiol 1989 Mar;63(10):114E–20E.

Fiebach N, Cook EF, Lee TH et al. Outcomes in patients with myocardial infarction who are initially admitted to stepdown units: data from the Multicenter Chest Pain Study. Am J Med 1990;89:15–20.

Feinleib M. Epidemiologic evidence for cardiovascular disease initiatives in Israel and the United States. Public Health Rep 1984 May;99(3):248–55.

Feinleib M, Havlik RJ, Gillum RF et al. Coronary heart disease and related procedures. National Hospital Discharge Survey data. Circulation 1989 Jun;79(6 Pt 2):113–8.

Figueras J, Lidon R, Cortadellas J. Rebound myocardial ischaemia following abrupt interruption of intravenous nitroglycerin infusion in patients with unstable angina at rest. Eur Heart J 1991 Mar;12:405–11.

Fineberg HV, Scadden D, Goldman L. Care of patients with a low probability of acute myocardial infarction. Cost effectiveness of alternatives to coronary-care-unit admission. N Engl J Med 1984 May;310:1301–7.

Freeman MR, Langer A, Wilson RF et al. Thrombolysis in unstable angina. Randomized double-blind trial of t-PA and placebo. Circulation 1992 Jan;85(1):150–7.

Fuster V, Badimon L, Badimon JJ et al. The pathogenesis of coronary artery disease and the acute coronary syndromes (2). N Engl J Med 1992 Jan;326(5):310–8.

Gerstenblith G, Ouyang P, Achuff SC et al. Nifedipine in unstable angina: A double-blind randomized trial. N Engl J Med 1982 Apr;306(15):885–9.

Ghali JK, Cooper RS, Kowatly I et al. Delay between onset of chest pain and arrival to the coronary care unit among minority and disadvantaged patients. J Natl Med Assoc 1993 Mar;85:180–4.

Gibson RS, Beller GA, Gheorghiade M et al. The prevalence and clinical significance of residual myocardial ischemia 2 weeks after uncomplicated non-Q wave infarction: a prospective natural history study. Circulation 1986;73(6):1186–98.

Gibson RS, Young PM, Boden WE et al. Prognostic significance and beneficial effect of diltiazem on the incidence of early recurrent ischemia after non-Q-wave myocardial infarction: results from the Multicenter Diltiazem Reinfarction Study. Am J Cardiol 1987 Aug;60:203–9.

Gillum RF, Feinleib M. Coronary heart disease in the elderly. Compr Ther 1988 Aug;14(8):66–73.

Goldman L, Cook EF, Brand DA et al. A computer protocol to predict myocardial infarction in emergency department patients with chest pain. N Engl J Med 1988 Mar; 318(13):797–803.

Goldman L, Weinberg M, Weisberg M et al. A computer-derived protocol to aid in the diagnosis of emergency room patients with acute chest pain. N Engl J Med 1982; 307:588–96.

Gore JM, Goldberg RJ, Matsumoto AS et al. Validity of serum total cholesterol level obtained within 24 hours of acute myocardial infarction. Am J Cardiol 1984 Oct; 54:722–5.

Gortner SR, Gilliss CL, Paul SM et al. Expected and realized benefits from cardiac surgery: an update. Cardiovasc Nurs 1989 Jul;25(4):19–24.

Gottlieb SO, Weisfeldt ML, Ouyang P et al. Effect of the addition of propranolol to therapy with nifedipine for unstable angina pectoris: a randomized, double-blind, placebo-controlled trial. Circulation 1986 Feb;73(2):331–7.

Grambow DW, Topol EJ. Effect of maximal medical therapy on refractoriness of unstable angina pectoris. Am J Cardiol 1992 Sep;70:577–81.

Graves EJ. National hospital discharge survey: annual summary, 1991. National Center for Health Statistics. Vital Health Statistics. Series 13, Number 114. Washington: Public Health Service, 1993.

■ Grijseels EW, et al. Pre-hospital triage of patients with suspected myocardial infarction. Evaluation of previously developed algorithms and new proposals. Euro Hrt J 1995 16:325–32.

■ Hamm CW, Reimers J, et al. For the German Angioplasty Bypass Surgery Investigation: A randomized study of coronary angioplasty compared with bypass surgery in patients with symptomatic multivessel coronary disease. N Engl J Med 1994 331:1037–1043.

Hargarten KM, Aprahamian C, Stueven HA et al. Prophylactic lidocaine in the prehospital patient with chest pain of suspected cardiac origin. Ann Emer Med 1986 Aug;15(8):881–5.

Hargarten KM, Chapman PD, Stueven HA et al. Prehospital prophylactic lidocaine does not favorably affect outcome in patients with chest pain. Ann Emer Med 1990 Nov;19(11):1274–9.

Held PH, Yusuf S, Furberg C. Calcium channel blockers in acute myocardial infarction and unstable angina: an overview. Br Med J 1989 Nov;299:1187–92.

Heston TF, Lewis LM. Gender bias in the evaluation and management of acute nontraumatic chest pain. The St Louis Emergency Physicians' Association Research Group. Fam Prac Res J 1992 Dec;12:383–9.

Hirsh J. Heparin. N Engl J Med 1991;324:565–74.

■ Hussain KM, et al. Pacing-induced ST segment deviation in patients with unstable angina: clinical, angiographic, and hemodynamic correlation. Angiology 1995 46:567–76(A).

■ Hussain KM, et al. Unstable angina of crescendo pattern vs. new onset: a clinical, coronary arteriographic and hemodynamic study. Angiology 1995 46(6):497–502(B).

ISIS-2 (Second International Study of Infarct Survival) Collaborative Group. Randomized trial of intravenous streptokinase, oral aspirin, both, or neither among 17,187 cases of suspected acute myocardial infarction: ISIS-2. Lancet 1988 Aug;2(8607):349–60.

Jayes RL, Beshansky JR, D'Agostino RB et al. Do patients' coronary risk factor reports predict acute cardiac ischemia in the emergency department? J Clin Epidemiol 1992;45:621–6.

Kantrowitz A, Wasfie T, Freed PS et al. Intraaortic balloon pumping 1967 through 1982: analysis of complications in 733 patients. Am J Cardiol 1986 Apr;57:976–83.

Kaplan K, Davison R, Parker M et al. Intravenous nitroglycerin for the treatment of angina at rest unresponsive to standard nitrate therapy. Am J Cardiol 1983 Mar;51(5):694–8.

Karlson BW, Herlitz J, Pettersson P et al. A one-year prognosis in patients hospitalized with a history of unstable angina pectoris. Clin Cardiol 1993 May;16:397–402.

Karlsson JE, Berglund U, Bjorkholm A et al. Thrombolysis with recombinant human tissue-type plasminogen activator during instability in coronary artery disease: effect on myocardial ischemia and need for coronary revascularization. TRIC Study Group. Am Heart J 1992 Dec;124(6):1419–26.

Katus HA, Yasuda T, Gold HK et al. Diagnosis of acute myocardial infarction by detection of circulating cardiac myosin light chains. Am J Cardiol 1984 Nov;54:964–70.

■ King SB III, Lembo NJ, et al. For the emory angioplasty versus surgery trial (EAST): a randomized trial comparing coronary angioplasty with bypass surgery. N Engl J Med 1994 331:1044–1050.

Krone RJ, Dwyer EM, Greenberg H et al. Risk stratification in patients with first non-Q wave infarction: limited value of the early low level exercise test after uncomplicated infarcts. J Am Coll Cardiol 1989;14(1):31–7.

Larsson H, Areskog M, Areskog NH et al. Should the exercise test (ET) be performed at discharge or one month later after an episode of unstable angina or non-Q-wave myocardial infarction? Int J Card Imaging 1991;7(1):7–14.

Larsson H, Jonasson T, Ringqvist I et al. Diagnostic and prognostic importance of ST recording after an episode of unstable angina or non-Q-wave myocardial infarction. Eur Heart J 1992 Feb;13:207–12.

Lee TH, Cook EF, Weisberg M et al. Acute chest pain in the emergency room. Identification and examination of low-risk patients. Arch Intern Med 1985 Jan;145(1):65–9.

Lee TH, Cook EF, Weisberg MC et al. Impact of the availability of a prior electrocardiogram on the triage of the patient with acute chest pain. J Gen Intern Med 1990 Sep;5:381–8.

Lee TH, Goldman L. Serum enzyme assays in the diagnosis of acute myocardial infarction. Ann Intern Med 1986 Aug;105:221–33.

Lee TH, Juarez G, Cook EF et al. Ruling out acute myocardial infarction. A prospective multicenter validation of a 12-hour strategy for patients at low risk. N Engl J Med 1991 May;324(18):1239–46.

Lee TH, Weisberg MC, Brand DA et al. Candidates for thrombolysis among emergency room patients with acute chest pain: true and false positive rates. Ann Intern Med 1989 Jun;110:957–62.

Lewis HDJ, Davis JW, Archibald DG et al. Protective effects of aspirin against acute myocardial infarction and death in men with unstable angina. Results of a Veterans Administration Cooperative Study. N Engl J Med 1983 Aug;309(7):396–403.

■ Lindenfeld J and Morrison DA. Toward a stable clinical classification of unstable angina. J Am Coll Cardiol 1995 25:1293–94.

Lubsen J, Tijssen JG. Efficacy of nifedipine and metoprolol in the early treatment of unstable angina in the coronary care unit: findings from the Holland Interuniversity Nifedipine/metoprolol Trial (HINT). Am J Cardiol 1987 Jul;60(2):18A–25A.

Luchi RJ, Scott SM, Deupree RH. Comparison of medical and surgical treatment for unstable angina pectoris. Results of a Veterans Administration Cooperative Study. N Engl J Med 1987 Apr;316(16):977–84.

Madsen JK, Thomsen BL, Mellemgaard K et al. Independent prognostic risk factors for patients referred because of suspected acute myocardial infarction without confirmed diagnosis. Prognosis after discharge in relation to medical history and non-invasive investigations. Eur Heart J 1988;9(6):611–8.

Makhoul RG, Cole CW, McCann RL. Vascular complications of the intra-aortic balloon pump: an analysis of 436 patients. Am Surg 1993 Sep;59:564–8.

Mark DB, Califf R, Morris K, et al. Clinical characteristics and long-term survival of patients with variant angina. Circulation 1984;69:880–8.

Mark DB, Nelson CL, Califf RM et al. The continuing evolution of therapy for coronary artery disease: initial results from the era of coronary angioplasty. Circulation, 1994;89:2015–2025.

Mark DB, Shaw, L, Harrell FE et al. Prognostic value of a treadmill exercise score in outpatients with suspected coronary artery disease. N Engl J Med 1991 Sep;325:849–53.

Marmur JD, Freeman MR, Langer A et al. Prognosis in medically stabilized unstable angina: early Holter ST-segment monitoring compared with predischarge exercise thallium tomography. Ann Intern Med 1990 Oct;113:575–9.

May DC, Popma JJ, Black WH. In vivo induction and reversal of nitroglycerin tolerance in human coronary arteries. N Engl J Med 1987 Sep;317:805–9.

McCarthy BD, Beshansky JR, D'Agostino RB et al. Missed diagnoses of acute myocardial infarction in the emergency department: results from a multicenter study. Ann Emerg Med 1993 Mar;22(3):579–82.

McCarthy BD, Wong JB, Selker HP. Detecting acute cardiac ischemia in the emergency department: a review of the literature. J Gen Intern Med 1990 Jul;5:365–73.

McCormick JR, Schick ECJ, McCabe CH et al. Determinants of operative mortality and long-term survival in patients with unstable angina. The CASS experience. J Thorac Cardiovasc Surg 1985 May;89(5):683–8.

McNutt RA, Selker HP. How did the acute ischemic heart disease predictive instrument reduce unnecessary coronary care unit admissions? Med Decis Making 1988 Apr;8(2):90–4.

■ Mehran R, Ambrose A, et al. for the TAUSA Study Group. Angioplasty of complex lesions in ischemic rest angina: results of the thrombolysis and angioplasty in unstable angina (TAUSA) trial. J Am Coll Cardiol 1995 26:961–966.

Moise A, Theroux P, Taeymans Y et al. Clinical and angiographic factors associated with progression of coronary artery disease. J Am Coll Cardiol 1984 Mar;3(3):659–67.

■ Moreyra AE, et al. Coronary angioplasty in unstable angina; contemporary experience. Canadian J Card 1995 11:385–90.

■ Morrison DA, Sacks J, et al. Effectiveness of percutaneous transluminal coronary angioplasty for patients with medically refractory rest angina pectoris and high risk of adverse outcomes with coronary artery bypass grafting. Am J Cardiol 1995 75: 237–240.

Moss AJ, Goldstein RE, Hall WJ et al. Detection and significance of myocardial ischemia in stable patients after recovery from an acute coronary event. Multicenter Myocardial Ischemia Research Group. JAMA 1993 May;269:2379–85.

Muller JE, Turi ZG, Pearle DL et al. Nifedipine and conventional therapy for unstable angina pectoris: a randomized double-blind comparison. Circulation 1984 Apr; 69:728–39.

National Center for Health Statistics. Kozak LJ, Moien M. Detailed diagnoses and surgical procedures for patients discharged from short-stay hospitals. United States, 1983. Vital and Health Statistics, Series 12, No. 82 [DHHS Pub. No. (PHS) 85-1743]. Washington: Public Health Service, March 1985.

National Institute of Health. Recommendations for improving cholesterol measurement [NIH Pub. No. 90-2964]. Bethesda [MD]: National Heart, Lung, and Blood Institute, February 1990.

Nyman I, Areskog M, Areskog NH et al. Very early risk stratification by electrocardiogram at rest in men with suspected unstable coronary heart disease. J Intern Med 1993;234:293–301.

Nyman I, Larsson H, Areskog M et al. The predictive value of silent ischemia at an exercise test before discharge after an episode of unstable coronary artery disease. RISC Study Group. Am Heart J 1992 Feb;123(2):324–31.

Parisi AF, Folland ED, Hartigan P et al. A comparison of angioplasty with medical therapy in the treatment of single-vessel coronary artery disease. N Engl J Med 1992 Jan;326(1):10–6.

Parisi AF, Khuri S, Deupree RH et al. Medical compared with surgical management of unstable angina. 5-year mortality and morbidity in the Veterans Administration Study. Circulation 1989 Nov;80(5):1176–89.

Pozen MW, D'Agostino RB, Selker HP et al. A predictive instrument to improve coronary-care-unit admission practices in acute ischemic heart disease. A prospective multicenter clinical trial. N Engl J Med 1984 May;310(20):1273–8.

Pryor DB, Harrell FE, Lee KL et al. Estimating the likelihood of significant coronary artery disease. Am J Med 1983 Nov;75(5):771–80.

Pryor DB, Shaw L, McCants CB et al. Value of the history and physical in identifying patients at increased risk for coronary artery disease. Ann Intern Med 1993 Jan;118:81–90.

Rahimtoola SH, Nunley D, Grunkemeier G et al. Ten-year survival after coronary bypass surgery for unstable angina. N Engl J Med 1983 Mar;308(12):676–81.

Rankin JS, Newton JR Jr, Califf RM et al. Clinical characteristics and current management of medically refractory unstable angina. Ann Surg 1984 Oct;200:457–65.

Raschke RA, Reilly BM, Guidry JR et al. The weight-based heparin dosing nomogram compared with a "standard care" nomogram. Ann Intern Med 1993 Nov;119: 874–81.

Reichek N, Priest C, Zimrin D et al. Antianginal effects of nitroglycerin patches. Am J Cardiol 1984 Jul;54(1):1–7.

RISC Group. Risk of myocardial infarction and death during treatment with low dose aspirin and intravenous heparin in men with unstable coronary artery disease. Lancet 1990 Oct;336(8719):827–30.

RITA Trial Participants. Coronary angioplasty versus coronary artery bypass surgery: the Randomized Intervention Treatment of Angina (RITA) trial. Lancet 1993 Mar;341(8845):573–80.

Roberts KB, Califf RM, Harrell FE et al. The prognosis for patients with new-onset angina who have undergone cardiac catheterization. Circulation 1983 Nov;68(5):970–8.

Rouan GW, Lee TH, Cook EF et al. Clinical characteristics and outcome of acute myocardial infarction in patients with initially normal or nonspecific electrocardiograms (a report from the multicenter chest pain study). Am J Cardiol 1989;64:1087–92.

Roubin GS, Harris PJ, Eckhardt I et al. Intravenous nitroglycerine in refractory unstable angina pectoris. Aust N Z J Med 1982 Dec;12(6):598–602.

Russell RO, Moraski RE, Kouchoukos N et al. Unstable angina pectoris: National cooperative study group to compare surgical and medical therapy. Am J Cardiol 1978 Nov;42:839–48.

■ Salahas A, et al. Correlation of clinical and electrocardiography variables with coronary lesions in unstable angina pectoris. Angiology 1995 46:827–32.

Saran RK, Bhandari K, Narain VS et al. Intravenous streptokinase in the management of a subset of patients with unstable angina: a randomized controlled trial. Int J Cardiol 1990 Aug;28(2):209–13.

■ Savonitto S, et al. Combination therapy with metoprolol and nifedipine versus monotherapy in patients with stable angina pectoris. J Am Coll Cardiol 1996 27:311–16.

Sawe U. Early diagnosis of acute myocardial infarction with special reference to the diagnosis of the intermediate coronary syndrome: a clinical study. Acta Med Sci 1972;520(suppl):1–76.

Schechtman KB, Capone RJ, Kleiger RE et al. Risk stratification of patients with non-Q wave myocardial infarction. The critical role of ST segment depression. The Diltiazem Reinfarction Study Research Group. Circulation 1989 Nov;80:1148–58.

Schreiber TL, Rizik D, White C et al. Randomized trial of thrombolysis versus heparin in unstable angina. Circulation 1992 Nov;86(5):1407–14.

Schroeder JS, Lamb I, Hu M et al. Coronary bypass surgery for unstable angina pectoris. Long-term survival and function. JAMA 1977 Jun;237:2609–12.

Scott J, Huskisson EC. Graphic representation of pain. Pain 1976;2:175–84.

■ Scott SM, et al. VA study of unstable angina. 10-year results show duration of surgical advantage for patients with impaired ejection fraction. Circulation 1994 90: II120–3.

Scott SM, Luchi RJ, Deupree RH. Veterans Administration Cooperative Study for treatment of patients with unstable angina. Results in patients with abnormal left ventricular function. Circulation 1988 Sep;78(3 Pt 2):I113–21.

Selker HP, Griffith JL, D'Agostino RB. A tool for judging coronary care unit admission appropriateness, valid for both real-time and retrospective use. A time-sensitive predictive instrument (TIPI) for acute cardiac ischemia: a multicenter study. Med Care 1991;29:610–27.

Severi S, Orsini E, Marraccini P et al. The basal electrocardiogram and the exercise stress test in assessing prognosis in patients with unstable angina. Eur Heart 1988;9(4):441–6.

Sharma GV, Deupree RH, Khuri SF et al. Coronary bypass surgery improves survival in high-risk unstable angina. Results of a Veterans Administration Cooperative study with an 8-year follow-up. Veterans Administration Unstable Angina Cooperative Study Group. Circulation 1991 Nov;84(5 Suppl):III260–7.

SHEP Cooperative Research Group. Prevention of stroke by antihypertensive drug treatment in older persons with isolated systolic hypertension. Final results of the Systolic Hypertension in the Elderly Program (SHEP). JAMA 1991 Jun;265(24):3255–64.

Sherman CT, Litvack F, Grundfest W et al. Coronary angioscopy in patients with unstable angina pectoris. N Engl J Med 1986 Oct;315:913–9.

Silva P, Galli M, Campolo L. Prognostic significance of early ischemia after acute myocardial infarction in low-risk patients. IRES (Ischemia Residua) Study Group. Am J Cardiol 1993 May;71:1142–7.

Sriwatanakul K, Kelvie W, Lasagna L et al. Studies with different types of visual analog scales for measurement of pain. Clin Pharmacol Ther 1983 Aug;34(2):234–9.

Swahn E, Areskog M, Berglund U et al. Predictive importance of clinical findings and a pre-discharge exercise test in patients with suspected unstable coronary artery disease. Am J Cardiol 1987;59(4):208–14.

Telford AM, Wilson C. Trial of heparin versus atenolol in prevention of myocardial infarction in intermediate coronary syndrome. Lancet 1981 Jun;1(8232):1225–8.

Thadani U, Hamilton SF, Olsen E et al. Transdermal nitroglycerin patches in angina pectoris. Dose titration, duration of effect, and rapid tolerance. Ann Intern Med 1986 Oct;105(4):485–92.

Theroux P, Ouimet H, McCans J et al. Aspirin, heparin, or both to treat acute unstable angina. N Engl J Med 1988 Oct;319(17):1105–11.

Theroux P, Taeymans Y, Morissette D et al. A randomized study comparing propranolol and diltiazem in the treatment of unstable angina. J Am Coll Cardiol 1985 Mar;5(3):717–22.

Theroux P, Waters D, Lam J et al. Reactivation of unstable angina after the discontinuation of heparin. N Engl J Med 1992 Jul;327(3):141–5.

Theroux P, Waters D, Qiu S et al. Aspirin versus heparin to prevent myocardial infarction during the acute phase of unstable angina. Circulation 1993 Nov;88(part 1):2045–8.

Tierney WM, Roth BJ, Psaty B et al. Predictors of myocardial infarction in emergency room patients. Crit Care Med 1985 Jul;13(7):526–31.

TIMI Study Group. The thrombolysis in myocardial infarction (TIMI) trial. N Engl J Med 1985 Apr;312(14):932–6.

TIMI IIIA Investigators. Early effects of tissue-type plasmogen activator added to conventional therapy on the culprit coronary lesion in patients presenting with ischemic cardiac pain at rest. Circulation 1993 Jan;87:38–52.

The TIMI IIIB Investigators: Effects of tissue plasminogen activator and a comparison of early invasive and conservative strategies in unstable and non-Q wave myocardial infarction. Results of the TIMI IIIB Trial. Circulation 1994 89:1545–1556.

Van der Does E, Lubsen J, Pool J et al. Acute coronary events in a general practice: objectives and design of the Imminent Myocardial Infarction Rotterdam Study. Heart Bull 1976;7:91–8.

■ Van Miltenburg AJM, et al. Incidence and follow-up of Braunwald subgroups in unstable angina pectoris. J Am Coll Cardiol 1995 25:1286–92.

Wallentin LC. Aspirin (75 mg/day) after an episode of unstable coronary artery disease: long-term effects on the risk for myocardial infarction, occurrence of severe angina and the need for revascularization. Research Group on Instability in Coronary Artery Disease in Southeast Sweden. J Am Coll Cardiol 1991 Dec;18(7):1587–93.

Wasson JH, Sox HC, Neff RK et al. Clinical prediction rules. Applications and methodological standards. N Engl J Med 1985 Sep;313(13):793–9.

Waters DD, Miller DD, Szlachcic J et al. Factors influencing the long-term prognosis of treated patients with variant angina. Circulation 1983 Aug;68(2):258–65.

Wears RL, Li S, Hernandez JD et al. How many myocardial infarctions should we rule out? Ann Emer Med 1989 Sep;18:953–63.

■ Weingarten SR, et al. Practice guidelines and reminders to reduce duration of hospital stay for patients with chest pain. Ann Intern Med 1994 120:257–263.

White LD, Lee TH, Cook EF et al. Comparison of the natural history of new onset and exacerbated chronic ischemic heart disease. The Chest Pain Study Group. J Am Coll Cardiol 1990 Aug;16(2):304–10.

Wilcox I, Freedman SB, McCredie RJ et al. Risk of adverse outcome in patients admitted to the coronary care unit with suspected unstable angina pectoris. Am J Cardiol 1989 Oct;64(14):845–8.

Williams DO, Kirby MG, McPherson K et al. Anticoagulant treatment of unstable angina. Br J Clin Prac 1986 Mar;40(3):114–6.

Young GP, Hedges JR, Gibler WB et al. Do CK-MB results affect chest pain decision making in the emergency department? Ann Emer Med 1991 Nov;20:1220–8.

Younis LT, Byers S, Shaw L et al. Prognostic value of intravenous dipyridamole thallium scintigraphy after an acute myocardial ischemic event. Am J Cardiol 1989;64(3):161–6.

Yusuf S, Collins R, MacMahon S et al. Effect of intravenous nitrates on mortality in acute myocardial infarction: an overview of the randomized trials. Lancet 1988 May;1(8594):1088–92.

Yusuf S, Pepine CJ, Garces C et al. Effect of enalapril on myocardial infarction and unstable angina in patients with low ejection fractions. Lancet 1992 Nov 14;340(8829):1173–8.

Yusuf S, Wittes J, Friedman L. Overview of results of randomized clinical trials in heart disease. II. Unstable angina, heart failure, primary prevention with aspirin, and risk factor modification. JAMA 1988 Oct;260(15):2259–63.

Zhu YY, Chung WS, Botvinick EH et al. Dipyridamole perfusion scintigraphy: The experience with its application in one hundred seventy patients with known or suspected unstable angina. Am Heart J 1991 Jan;121:33–43.

Glossary

Acute myocardial infarction: An acute process of myocardial ischemia with sufficient severity and duration to result in permanent myocardial damage.

Angina pectoris: A clinical syndrome typically characterized by a deep, poorly localized chest or arm discomfort that is reproducibly associated with physical exertion or emotional stress and relieved promptly by rest or sublingual NTG. The discomfort of angina is often hard for patients to describe, and many patients do not consider it to be "pain." Patients with unstable angina may have discomfort with all the qualities of typical angina except that episodes are more severe and prolonged and may occur at rest with an unknown relationship to exertion or stress. In most, but not all, patients these symptoms reflect myocardial ischemia resulting from significant underlying coronary artery disease. (CAD).

Angiographically significant CAD: CAD is typically judged "significant" at coronary angiography if there is at least a 70 percent diameter stenosis of one or more major epicardial coronary segments or at least a 50 percent diameter stenosis of the left main coronary artery. The term "significant CAD" used in this guideline does not imply clinical significance but refers only to an angiographically significant stenosis.

Anxiolytic therapy: Treatment to counteract or diminish anxiety.

Aortic stenosis: Narrowing of the aorta or its orifice usually due to disease of the valve.

Arrhythmia: Irregularity or loss of rhythm of the heartbeat.

Atherosclerosis: Nodular thickening or hardening of the layers in the wall of an artery; characterized by irregularly distributed lipid deposits in the intima of large and medium-sized arteries.

133

Beta blocker (β-adrenergic blocking agent): A drug that blocks the effect of catecholamines, producing a decrease in heart rate and oxygen demand in the myocardium.

Calcium antagonist: A drug that blocks entry of calcium into cells and inhibits the contractility of smooth muscle. The result is dilation of the blood vessels and a reduction in blood pressure.

Cardiac catheterization: Passage of a catheter into the heart through a blood vessel leading to the heart for the purpose of measuring intracardiac pressure abnormalities, obtaining cardiac blood samples, and/or imaging cardiac structures by injection of radio-opaque dye.

Cardiac mortality: Death due to cardiac cause.

Cardiopulmonary resuscitation: An emergency measure to maintain a person's breathing and heartbeat when they have stopped as a result of myocardial infarction, trauma, or other disorder.

Cardiogenic shock: Failure to maintain blood supply to the tissues because of inadequate cardiac output, such as may be caused in myocardial infarction.

Chronic obstructive pulmonary disease: A group of conditions in which the patient has an expiratory airflow obstruction such as chronic bronchitis or emphysema.

Comorbidity: A concomitant but unrelated pathologic or disease process, usually used to indicate coexistence of two or more disease processes.

Congestive heart failure: Failure of the heart to maintain adequate circulation of blood.

Coronary artery bypass grafting: Vein or artery grafted surgically to permit blood to travel from the aorta to a branch of the coronary artery at a point past an obstruction.

Coronary artery disease (CAD): Although a number of disease processes other than atherosclerosis can involve coronary arteries, in this guideline the term CAD refers to the atherosclerotic narrowing of the major epicardial coronary arteries.

Coronary stenosis: Narrowing or constriction of any orifices leading into or from the heart or between chambers of the heart.

Coronary thrombus: A blood clot that obstructs a blood vessel of the heart.

Echocardiography: Use of ultrasound in the investigation of the heart and great vessels and diagnosis of cardiovascular lesions.

Ejection fraction: The percent of blood emptied from the ventricle by the end of a contraction of the heart.

Exercise tolerance testing: Also referred to as a stress test, a diagnostic test in which the patient exercises on a treadmill, bicycle, or other equipment while heart activity is monitored by an ECG.

Hemodynamic instability: Instability of the blood pressure.

Hypercholesterolemia: Excessive cholesterol in the blood.

Hyperlipidemia: Excessive quantity of fat (cholesterol and triglycerides) in the blood.

Hypertrophic cardiomyopathy: Disease of the myocardium produced by the enlargement of the cells of the myocardium; often the result of increased oxygen demand in ischemic heart disease.

Hypotension: Decrease of systolic and diastolic blood pressure below normal.

Intra-aortic balloon pump: Use of a balloon attached to a catheter inserted through the femoral artery into the descending thoracic aorta for producing alternating inflation and deflation during diastole and systole, respectively.

Intracoronary stenting: Use of a prosthetic metal device to provide and maintain an enlarged coronary lumen at the side of an obstructive atherosclerotic plaque.

Ischemic heart disease: A form of heart disease whose primary manifestations result from myocardial ischemia due to atherosclerotic CAD. This term encompasses a spectrum of patients ranging from the asymptomatic preclinical phase to acute myocardial infarction and sudden cardiac death.

Left bundle branch block: An ECG change characterized by an intraventricular conduction delay affecting the left ventricular wall and septum. Acute occurrences most commonly result from myocardial ischemia.

Left ventricular function: Function of the main pumping chamber of the heart that receives blood from the left atrium and pumps it out into the general circulation through the aortic valve.

Left main disease: Stenosis of the left main coronary artery.

Likelihood: Used in this guideline to refer to the probability of an underlying diagnosis, particularly significant CAD.

Mitral regurgitation: Abnormal systolic back flow of blood from the left ventricle into the left atrium, resulting from imperfect closure of the mitral valve.

Myocardial infarction (MI): Damage to the heart muscle caused by occlusion of one or more of the coronary arteries.

Myocardial ischemia: A condition in which oxygen delivery to and waste removal from the myocardium falls below normal levels with oxygen demand exceeding supply. As a consequence, the metabolic machinery of myocardial cells is impaired leading to various degrees of systolic (contractile) and diastolic (relaxation) dysfunction. Ischemia is usually diagnosed indirectly through techniques that demonstrate reduced myocardial blood flow or its consequences on contracting myocardium.

Myocardium: The muscular wall of the heart located between the inner endocardial layer and the outer epicardial layer.

Multivessel disease: Indicates that two or more of the coronary arteries are diseased.

Nitrate: A drug whose metabolites produce a relaxation of vascular smooth muscle. This in turn produces a strong dilation of the veins, reducing preload and myocardial oxygen demand.

Non-Q-wave myocardial infarction: An acute myocardial infarction that is not associated with the evolution of new Q-waves on the ECG. The diagnosis of non-Q-wave myocardial infarction is often difficult to make soon after the event and is commonly made only retrospectively on the basis of elevated cardiac enzyme levels.

Percutaneous transluminal coronary angioplasty (PTCA): A method of treating localized coronary artery narrowing using a special catheter with a cylindrical balloon surrounding it that can be inflated to dilate the narrowed vessel.

Perfusion balloon angioplasty: A variation of PTCA in which a catheter is inserted in the artery that permits blood flow during balloon inflation.

Perfusion scan: A test to determine the status of blood flow to an organ.

Pharmacologic stress test: A test of heart function during intentional drug-induced stress.

Post-MI angina: Unstable angina occurring from 1 to 60 days after an acute MI.

Pulmonary edema: A condition, usually acute, but sometimes chronic, where fluid builds up in the lungs. This often occurs as a response to left ventricular failure in ischemic heart disease, hypertension, or aortic valve disease.

Radionuclide test: A diagnostic test in which a radioactive substance is injected into the bloodstream and the emitted radioactivity is detected by a scanner; used to visualize the heart and vessels.

Reperfusion-eligible acute myocardial infarction: A condition characterized by a clinical presentation compatible with acute myocardial infarction accompanied by ST-segment elevation or left bundle branch block on ECG.

Restenosis: The recurrence of a stenosis in a coronary artery.

Revascularization: Restoration, to the extent possible, of normal blood flow to the myocardium by surgical or percutaneous means or with removal or reduction of an obstruction as occurs when CABG or PTCA is performed.

Risk: High, intermediate, and low risk in this guideline refer to the probability of future adverse cardiac events, particularly death or MI.

Sinus node rate: Under normal conditions, the pacemaker function of the heart resides in the sinus node; normal heart rate.

Stenosis: A narrowing or blockage of a coronary artery.

Sublingual: Beneath the tongue.

Supraventricular arrhythmia: An irregular heart beat that originates in the atria or AV node.

Thrombocytopenia: Abnormal decrease in number of the blood platelets.

Thrombolytic therapy: Pharmacologic treatment with a class of drugs that can break up fibrin blood clots.

Transvenous pacemaker: Cardiac pacemaker using a pacing electrode or wire passed through a vein into the chambers of the heart that stimulates and maintains a normal heart rate; may be permanent or temporary.

Triage: Screening and classification of sick, wounded, or injured persons to determine priority of need and proper place of treatment.

Unstable angina: Chest pain that occurs at rest, new onset of pain with exertion, or pain that has accelerated (more frequent, longer in duration, or lower in threshold).

Variant angina: A clinical syndrome of rest pain and reversible ST-segment elevation without subsequent enzyme evidence of acute MI. In some patients, the cause of this syndrome appears to be coronary vasospasm alone often at the site of an insignificant coronary plaque, but a majority of patients with variant angina have angiographically significant CAD.

Ventriculography: A procedure for visualization of ventricles of the heart by x-ray after injection of a contrast material.

Acronyms

ACLS	Advanced cardiac life support
ACME	Angioplasty Compared with Medicine [study]
ADP	Adenosine diphosphate
AHCPR	Agency for Health Care Policy and Research
aPTT	Activated partial thromboplastin time
ASA	Aspirin
AV	Atrioventricular
BB	Brain
BLS	Basic life support
CABG	Coronary artery bypass graft
CABRI	Coronary Artery Bypass Revascularization Investigation
CAD	Coronary artery disease
CCSC	Canadian Cardiovascular Society Classification
CCU	Coronary care unit
CHF	Congestive heart failure
CI	Confidence interval
CK	Creatinine kinase
COPD	Chronic obstructive pulmonary disease
DUMC	Duke University Medical Center
EAST	Emory Angioplasty Study Trial
ECG	12-lead electrocardiogram
ED	Emergency department
EF	Ejection fraction [left ventricle]
EMT	Emergency medical transport
GAB	German Angioplasty Bypass Surgery Investigation

GI	Gastrointestinal
HDL	High-density lipoprotein
IABP	Intra-aortic balloon pump
ICU	Intensive care unit
IHD	Ischemic heart disease
IMIR	Imminent MI Rotterdam [criteria]
ISIS	International Study of Infarct Survival
IV	Intravenous
IVCD	Interventricular conduction defect
LAD	Left anterior descending coronary artery
LBBB	Left bundle branch block
LDH	Lactate dehydrogenase
LV	Left ventricular
MB	Cardiac muscle
MET	Metabolic equivalent
MI	Myocardial infarction
MM	Skeletal muscle
MR	Mitral regurgitation
NHLBI	National Heart, Lung, and Blood Institute
NTG	Nitroglycerin
PR	ECG PR segment
PTCA	Percutaneous transluminal coronary angioplasty
PTT	Partial thromboplastin time
PVD	Peripheral vascular disease
RISC	Research Group on Instability in Coronary Artery Disease
RITA	Randomized Intervention Treatment of Angina
SBP	Systolic blood pressure
TIMI	Thrombolysis in myocardial infarction
VA	Veterans Administration

Index